Advance Praise for
1001 Simple Ways to Lose Weight

"At last. Sensible strategies for weight management that really are simple and really do work."

> —John P. Foreyt, Ph.D., professor
> of medicine and psychology,
> director, Nutrition Research
> Clinic, Baylor College of
> Medicine, coauthor of *Living
> Without Dieting*

"Everything it took me years of struggle to learn in a single book. A remarkable achievement . . . It puts you in control, gives you practical direction, and even fills you with hope! Destined to have that well-worn, thumbed-through look of every useful book on your shelf."

> —Ann Daniels (lost 150 pounds
> seven years ago)

"I can't tell you how refreshing it is to read a truly honest weight-control book. This is a very helpful guide packed with simple tips you'll find useful in everyday life."

> —Maria Simonson, Ph.D., Sc.D.,
> professor of psychology, founder
> and director, Health, Weight &
> Stress Clinic, Johns Hopkins
> Medical Institutions

"This book has practical advice for doable things without gimmicks . . . good, easy-to-follow recommendations."

—Carlos Dujovne, M.D., professor of medicine, director, Lipid and Arteriosclerosis Prevention Clinic, University of Kansas School of Medicine, author of *A Change of Heart*; and Leslie Votaw, M.S., R.D.

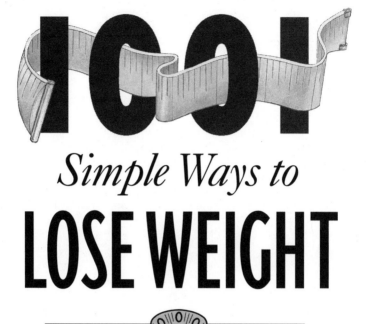

Simple Ways to
LOSE WEIGHT

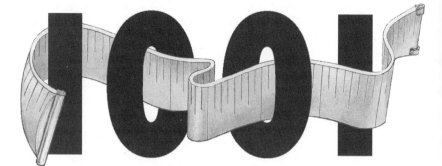

1001

Simple Ways to

LOSE WEIGHT

Proven Tips for Losing Those Extra Pounds—*and Keeping Them Off*

Gary L. Rempe

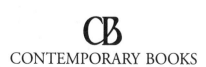

CONTEMPORARY BOOKS

Library of Congress Cataloging-in-Publication Data

Rempe, Gary L.
    1001 simple ways to lose weight : proven tips for losing those
extra pounds — and keeping them off / Gary L. Rempe.
       p.   cm.
    Includes bibliographical references.
    ISBN 0-8092-3080-1
    1. Weight loss.   I. Title.
RM222.2.R458   1997
613.2'5—dc20   96-47054
                                                   CIP

Cover design by Scott Rattray
Interior design by Mary Lockwood

1001 Simple Ways to Lose Weight is a trademark of Gary Rempe.

Published by Contemporary Books
A division of NTC/Contemporary Publishing Group, Inc.
4255 West Touhy Avenue, Lincolnwood (Chicago), Illinois 60712-1975 U.S.A.
Copyright © 1997 by Gary Rempe
Foreword © 1997 by Ann Daniels
Printed in the United States of America
International Standard Book Number: 0-8092-3080-1
00 01 02 03 04 05 ML 19 19 19 18 17 16 15 14 13 12 11 10 9 8 7 6 5 4

To Susan My Love

Contents

Author's Note

A s with any weight-control program or plan, you should obtain your physician's permission before and while following the menu plans, recipes, and advice in *1001 Simple Ways to Lose Weight*. This is absolutely necessary if you have a medical problem such as heart disease, high blood pressure, or diabetes. If you suffer from serious depression or high stress, you should consult with a psychologist or psychiatrist before following this book's advice. A registered dietician's help is also recommended.

Foreword

I t's hard for me to believe I've been asked to write a foreword for *1001 Simple Ways to Lose Weight*. You see, for 17 years I had no answers about effective weight loss. The nearly 300 pounds I carried on my five-foot two-inch frame was tragic proof I hadn't a clue about how to lose weight and keep it off.

Those who lacked tact asked how I managed to become so immense. The answer was simple. I believed in dieting and in losing weight as fast as humanly possible. At 12 years old, I began the nightmarish and all-too-common cycle of starting the latest diet, feeling deprived and miserable, then eating everything in sight. In the process I lost only one thing: self-esteem. This destructive diet/binge cycle continued for 17 painful years. Today I'm 150 pounds light and have been for seven years! I've been honored on the "Mike and Maty" talk show, and my story was featured in *Shape* magazine. I now help others lose weight by working with my local hospital, lecturing, and writing books.

You probably think the next sentence will read, "I finally lost weight when I gave up dieting." Yes, I did give up dieting, but more important, I decided I had to find my *own* answers to permanent weight loss. I had to find something that was comfortable for me, Ann Daniels, a person who would never look at a menu without reading the dessert section first. I made a conscious choice that I would be the one in control of my life.

I then began taking what I thought of as "baby steps" toward food control and healthy choices. My focus was on doing just a little better each day. At first this meant forgiving myself for eating something such as a cream-filled doughnut. I'd tell myself that eating one was better than devouring a whole box. In retrospect this might not seem like much, but it was progress. My self-confidence and self-esteem grew with each small success. What's more, these successes motivated me enough to continue to educate myself about what food choices worked for me. Eventually I found that the momentary pleasure of eating a doughnut wasn't worth the fat and calories that came with it, and I substituted foods that were healthier.

After a few months of concentrating on making many small food changes, it occurred to me that in my quest to lose weight I could eat more if I *moved* more. I'd honestly never thought of this before. I could never understand why anyone would want to exercise and sweat. How could sweating make anyone feel better? I couldn't imagine. If exercise meant I could eat more food, however, then surely it was worth a try.

Here again I began with baby steps. I took it very slowly and gradually increased my exercise each day. I also stopped focusing on the exercise I was performing and instead focused on how good I'd feel the next morning. The result is that I've exercised at least four days a week for the past nine years. Now I can't even begin to imagine giving up something that makes both my mind and body feel so terrific. This is remarkable when you consider I spent 40 years avoiding any kind of physical exertion!

While slowly changing my diet and exercise habits, I also learned to enjoy the entire process of losing weight. I focused on how I'd feel the next day when I awoke a little trimmer and healthier instead of impatiently waiting for the day I'd finally be thin. What a relief it was to allow myself to feel good for a change. It felt wonderful, and I began a productive cycle that lead to a 150-pound weight loss over a two-year period.

Since educating myself was the key to my success, I certainly wish I had had a book like *1001 Simple Ways to Lose Weight* nine years ago. It gives answers to each and every area with which I struggled. It provides practical solutions to all parts of the weight-loss puzzle using a delight-ful conversational style. Reading it is like talking to a knowledgeable and concerned friend, which is something that really would have helped me as I searched for answers. Its sensible approach counteracts the ineffective fast and superficial approaches many unscrupulous authors promote. It contains a unique and wonderful treasure trove of valuable tips that can benefit anyone who wants to lead a healthier life through better weight control.

Ann Daniels
(Lost 150 pounds seven years ago)

Preface

From tragic firsthand experience I knew at an early age that weight control is critical to good health. In my youth I arrived home from high school one day to find my 44-year-old father suffering a massive heart attack on our kitchen floor due to arteriosclerosis (clogged arteries). He miraculously pulled through but then still refused to stop eating high-fat foods and walk regularly for exercise. Consequently he suffered another massive heart attack several years later. Afterward he was expected to live only one or two years. At this point he finally started to walk each evening and reduce his fat and calorie intake. After a year of new healthier habits, his doctor, my family, and I couldn't believe the difference in his health. He not only substantially improved his poor cholesterol levels, but he also grew a network of new smaller arteries around his old clogged arteries! As I write this he's still alive and in good health.

From this early experience I learned that weight control, in the form of moderate exercise and dietary change, is important to our health. At the time, however, I didn't realize how an overweight condition can impact our lives beyond the threat of heart disease. After years of research I've firmly concluded that both our bodies and our minds can be profoundly affected by obesity. To illustrate, here's a list of ailments to which obesity can contribute:

Your Body

- Breast cancer
- Heart disease
- Stroke
- High blood pressure
- Diabetes mellitus
- Colon cancer
- Prostate cancer
- Cervical cancer
- Ovarian cancer
- Surgical complications
- Back pain
- Arthritis
- Hernias
- Hemorrhoids
- Gallbladder disease
- Breathing difficulties
- Sleeping disorders

Your Mind

- Low self-esteem
- Low self-confidence
- A sense of having no power
- Loneliness
- Moodiness
- Anger
- Inferiority complex
- Frustration
- Resentment
- Severe depression
- Self-hatred

Now you can understand why many physicians often end their check-ups by saying, "And you could also stand to lose a few pounds."

Equally alarming, however, is that the prevalence of obesity in America is growing at an astonishing rate. Today 33 percent of Americans are obese, compared with 24 percent just a decade ago! Among leading experts it's a well-known fact that obesity is one of the biggest health threats confronting people in affluent societies.

It's for these reasons, among others, that I spent the past five years researching and writing this quick-reference guidebook, despite the often overwhelming demands of four young children (two of whom were two-year-old twins!) and a wife with her own hectic career. I want you to have easy access to practical, quality information you can use in your daily life. Even if you made only a dozen or so of the ideas in this book a part of your everyday life, you would substantially improve your weight control. Take a minute to look through the following pages. You'll be glad you did!

If you have any questions, tips, or ideas you'd like to share, I'd be happy to here from you. Drop me a line at:

Seattle Institute for Weight Control Research
P.O. Box 51015
Seattle, WA 98115

Acknowledgments

First and foremost I want to thank my family: my beloved wife Susan who was always supportive; our two older children, Caroline and Philip, and my mother-in-law, Cheryl Ward, for doing far more than their share of baby-sitting; our twin toddlers, Gregory and Clara, for giving me many hours of smiles and laughter; my parents, Gary and Kathy, and my sister, Patience, for their heartfelt encouragement.

I want to thank one of the kindest people I've ever met, Constance Barthold, for her support of my work. Ann Daniels took time from her life to write a wonderful foreword for the book. She's an inspiration to everyone, and I feel privileged to know her. Thanks also go to my literary agent Jeff Herman for his time and expertise.

The study of overweight is such a large and complex field that it's impossible for a single person to write a comprehensive and accurate weight-control book without the help of many specialists. I am grateful to the following leading experts who took time out of their hectic schedules to share their expertise, time, and opinions: Carlos A. Dujovne, M.D., director of the Lipid and Arteriosclerosis Prevention Clinic at the University of Kansas School of Medicine, and Leslie Votaw, M.S., R.D.; John P. Foreyt, Ph.D., director of the Nutrition Research Clinic at the Baylor College of Medicine; Sachiko St. Jeor, Ph.D., R.D., director of the Nutrition and Education Program at the University of

Nevada School of Medicine; Alisa Minear, M.S., R.D., director of Nutrition and Health Education at the Scripps Clinic and Research Foundation; Maria Simonson, Ph.D., Sc.D., founder and director of the Health, Weight & Stress Clinic at Johns Hopkins Medical Institutions; and James Skinner, Ph.D., director of the Exercise and Sport Research Institute at Arizona State University.

Introduction

S usan Rempe permanently lost 34 pounds in just 18 weeks *after* having twins! As if losing weight and keeping it off after carrying two babies wasn't hard enough in itself, she also had to cope with the incredible demands of raising two older children and twin infants, getting a Ph.D. in chemistry, keeping her husband happy, and doing all of the countless other things you have to do every day of your life. A mother of four at 32 years of age, Susan is now five-feet seven-inches tall, 125 pounds, and solid muscle. How did she do it? Was she special? Was she naturally thin? Was it a miracle? No. Like me (I lost 30 pounds 10 years ago) and many of the people in the more than one thousand weight-control success stories I researched, Susan gradually made a number of small changes in her attitude, diet, and exercise, and her extra weight came off as a by-product of a healthier lifestyle.

It's the Little Simple Things That Help Most

The truth is, weight-control success in the real world is usually the result of making small, simple changes in your day-to-day life that work for you personally. This just makes good solid sense for three fascinating reasons. First, your extra weight is typically the final product of little errors you make that have big consequences over time. A business-person, for instance, could gain 50 pounds from the time he or she is

30 to the time he or she is 40 from nothing more than two or three alcoholic drinks per week! If that same person ate one too many Oreo cookies each day over the same period of time, he or she could gain another 50 pounds. Your extra weight sneaks up on you until one day you wake up, look in the mirror, and say the classic line, "How did I ever let myself get this way?" Consequently, a reliable and manageable way to lose weight is to identify the small errors in your everyday life and then eliminate or reverse them. By working on turning your small errors into small successes you'll heighten your self-confidence as you start to accumulate many small wins; motivate yourself as success at one small thing leads to success at another; be less likely to quit, since a single slipup won't undo your many small changes; and be more likely to maintain your healthy lifestyle, since habits acquired through small changes are deeply ingrained.[1]

Second, if a weight-control solution is simple, then it's much more likely to become a natural part of your everyday life. During a weight-control attempt you're reorienting your lifestyle. Obviously, complicated weight-control strategies are going to be very difficult to transform into daily habits. Strategies using complex scientific terms are almost useless on a daily basis and are sometimes nothing more than a scheme designed to inflate the author's credibility. For instance, one popular diet book author recently wrote:

> Six types of simple sugars are found in foods, and the monosaccharide glucose is one of these. Another monosaccharide is fructose, which gives fruits and fruit juices their sweet taste. Galactose, also a monosaccharide, is seldom found by itself in nature but is instead a part of lactose, a simple sugar in milk.[2]

---

[1] Regarding the book's major theme, I wish to credit Kelly D. Brownell, professor of psychology at Yale and codirector of the Yale Center for Eating and Weight Disorders, as the person who has promoted most widely the theory that "extra weight is the final result of many small behavioral acts." A study of people in a large Health Maintenance Organization published in the November 1990 issue of the *American Journal of Clinical Nutrition* is one of the best scientific studies that demonstrate that people who succeed at losing weight and keeping it off do so through small realistic changes.

[2] Cliff Sheats, *Lean Bodies* (New York: Warner Books, 1992), 43.

This kind of detailed information is fine for scientists, but how in the world are you going to use it in your daily life? Most of what you need to know about fruit in relation to good nutrition can be summarized in the single American Dietetic Association guideline "Consume two to four servings from the fruit group each day." This may not be complicated enough for some authors, but it's the truth and it's practical. In order for a weight-control solution to work in daily life, it must be simple to use.

Third, weight control is a personal experience that can vary dramatically from one person to another. Not long ago, an impressive study of people in a large HMO published in the *American Journal of Clinical Nutrition* demonstrated that people who adapt and develop their own weight-control solutions are most likely to lose their weight and keep it off. The striking characteristic shared by people who lose weight permanently is that, during the second or so week of their weight-control program when everyone else quits, they start to customize their programs to suit their own lifestyles! The product of their personal effort is final victory over their weight. There's no one almighty right way to lose weight. Anyone who tells you otherwise, whether it be a best friend, a leading scientist, a Hollywood star, or an employee at a commercial diet center, is misleading you. Professionals, support groups, family, and friends can be very helpful, but they're not *you*. The best advice they can give you is tips that worked for other people. It's then your responsibility to see if these tips might work for you as is, or with some changes. If you want to lose weight and keep it off, you have to discover what's best for you. You have to do it your way so that it's your plan and you're in control.

True experts agree, and you probably already know, that to lose weight permanently you need to be more active and consume fewer calories and fat grams. What isn't widely known, however, is exactly *how* to make these general guidelines a natural part of our day-to-day lives by eliminating the many small errors we regularly make. After five years of intensive research, there's finally a real solution in *1001 Simple Ways to Lose Weight*. It's the first and only guidebook to identify these small choices, and then to provide hundreds of practical, simple tips anyone can use to make the right choices. The revolutionary result is a quick-reference guidebook that enables you to customize your weight control by picking and choosing, from 1,001 simple tips, the solutions that work best for you.

You can think of weight control as a complex gourmet dish. If you just look at it as a whole, then successfully preparing it seems very complicated indeed. If, however, someone breaks the dish down into the many small steps it takes to prepare it, then suddenly it isn't so complicated after all. This is what I've done with *1001 Simple Ways to Lose Weight*. I took the complicated process of weight control, broke it down into its many small parts, and then created simple, concise solutions you can try to make all of these small parts fit together for you personally.

The North American Weight-Control Survey

To create this potpourri of proven ideas, more than one thousand weight-control success stories from people across North America were used. Who could know more about the experience of losing weight than real people who actually did it? These stories of weight-loss winners were accumulated and studied as part of the Seattle Institute's unique North American Weight-Control Survey, the largest survey of proven success stories ever undertaken. The focus of this five-year non-scientific survey was to determine exactly what specific strategies people used who actually lost weight and kept it off.[3] Ideas culled from this survey were then combined with the newest scientific discoveries in psychology, diet, and exercise to create the smorgasbord of proven advice you'll find throughout *1001 Simple Ways to Lose Weight*. This combination of real-life successes and scientific facts gives you the best of both worlds and the largest variety of simple weight-control solutions possible.

[3]By "nonscientific" I mean the success stories that were used didn't lend themselves to statistical analysis. Each success story studied, however, did have before-and-after photographs for proof of weight loss, was part of published scientific research, or was published in a national periodical. If you'd like to read some of these success stories yourself, you'll find information in the "Suggested Readings" section at the end of this book.

How to Do It in the Real World

The practical guidebook approach of *1001 Simple Ways to Lose Weight* goes beyond that taken by most diet books. Diet books provide you with limited formulas to control your weight, without giving you the real-life solutions needed to make the diet a natural part of your everyday life. Obviously, trendy diet books that state you should consume mainly grapefruit, or maybe avocados, or perhaps hard candy fail to help you. But even a truthful diet book, based on the accurate premise that you need to eat more complex carbohydrates (i.e., breads, pastas, grains) and less fat, will fail to help you if you find yourself unable to apply its advice in your daily life. "Transition diets" that are less restrictive than the primary diet and some recipes near the back of the book are not enough. You need answers to crucial basic questions such as, How can you find more time for weight control? How do you cope with family and friends who eat fatty foods in front of you? What do you do when you arrive at a grocery store starving and loaded with money? What can you do to pinpoint quickly the cause of your binge? What can you do when you don't want to exercise? How do you deal with a jealous spouse? and How can you control your sampling when you prepare your meals? By dedicating the majority of its content to answering these and hundreds of other practical questions, *1001 Simple Ways to Lose Weight* will give you the real-world answers you've been searching for.

Part I features a new 7-step weight-control plan that's reliable, flexible, and easy to follow. Part II contains 1,001 simple tips designed to make the eating and exercise guidelines discussed in Part I fit naturally into your daily lifestyle. Read on, and take your first simple steps toward a healthier and happier life!

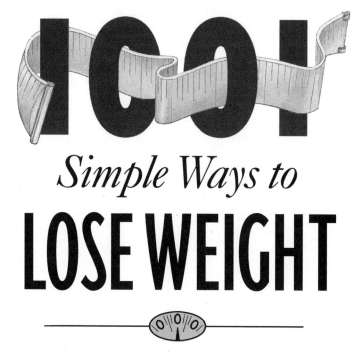

1001
Simple Ways to
LOSE WEIGHT

part one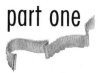

The Life Choice
7-Step Weight-Control Plan

Step 1.

Choose a Starting Place That's Right for You

There are four approaches from which you can choose to start your weight loss. The first is called the Small Changes Approach and is for people who are fed up with menu plans and diets that tell you exactly what to eat and drink. It's an easy and reliable approach that will help you structure a customized weight-control plan that works for you, and it's discussed next. The second approach is called the Real-Life Menu Exchange and is for people who do better on a program that initially limits choices, requires no calorie or fat-gram counting, and allows you to lose some weight quickly so that you're motivated to continue. It's presented in detail in Appendix A. The third approach is called the 10-Day Menu Exchange for a Hectic Life and is for people leading unusually busy lives. You'll find it in Appendix B. It's a short-term tool that can be used at the start of your weight-control effort, or anytime you don't want to cook. The fourth approach is called the Sensible Lifestyle Approach. It's a basic common-sense approach to healthy eating and smart exercise suitable for people who want the most freedom possible during weight loss and is discussed in Appendix C.

Take some time to read and think carefully about these approaches before you choose. As you ponder which approach you want to try first, you should also assess your motivation level. If you aren't bursting with enthusiasm to control your weight as you read this, then take a minute to read Tip 865. It contains a proven strategy that will help you decide whether or not you're motivated enough to start a weight-control program at this particular moment in your life.

The Small Changes Approach

Counting fat grams while on a low-fat diet is the most reliable way to lose weight, right? *Wrong!* Five years ago it was true that many people could consume almost all the nonfat foods they wanted and lose weight on a low-fat diet by keeping track of only fat grams. Older low-fat diet books such as Martin Katahn's *The T-Factor Diet* could even get away with making such bold proclamations as, "Note that some foods have so little fat that they can be eaten in unlimited quantities at any time, as part of your meals or as unlimited snacks."[4] Try following this advice today and you'll gain 10 pounds in the first two weeks alone. What Martin Katahn, Dean Ornish, Susan Powter, Covert Bailey, Cliff Sheats, and other major proponents of these older low-fat diets couldn't foresee was the unprecedented explosion of new nonfat processed food products that would burst into American supermarkets during the early 1990s. Since 1989 well over two thousand new low-fat processed foods, including everything from fat-free ham to ice cream and potato chips, have appeared on supermarket shelves. This has dramatically changed our food choices and, in the process, has made the older low-fat diets obsolete.

The words "fat free" and "nonfat" have actually become triggers that can cause overeating in many people! Personally, I have to make a conscious effort not to eat an extra serving or two when I see the words "fat free" on a package. It's easy to forget that just because something is fat free, that doesn't mean it's calorie free. Low-fat diets were a major breakthrough and do have many positive attributes. They lower your risk for health problems caused by too much dietary fat, and they can reduce feelings of deprivation during weight loss by allowing you to consume more calories than you could on a low-calorie diet. As researchers at Penn State University recently demonstrated, however, the

[4]Martin Katahn, *The T-Factor Diet*, revised edition (New York: Bantam, 1994), 32.

tragic flaw with low-fat diets today is that people cut their fat intake but still consume too many calories and so don't lose weight. This 7-step plan eliminates this problem by taking the much more reliable approach of keeping tabs on calories while you consume a healthy and satisfying low-fat diet.

Start by double-checking to ensure you're currently maintaining or losing your weight. You could track your weight for 7 to 10 days if you feel you need to. Ignore the daily fluctuations that almost everyone experiences. If you're within two pounds of your starting weight at the end of your test period, then you can proceed with your goal being to lose weight. If you're not within two pounds of your starting weight, then you'll have to start off with your goal being to reach weight maintenance; once you're able to maintain your weight, then you can start losing.

Now that you know whether your first goal is to lose weight or reach weight maintenance, pick a *typical weekday* (if you're female, this day should not be during menstruation) and honestly count how many calories you consume that day using food labels or a comprehensive calorie and fat guide and the form in Appendix D. Tips for using all of the form will be discussed in Step 4. For now, use it to count just calories. If you don't already have a calorie and fat guide, Karen J. Bellerson's *The Complete and Up-to-Date Fat Book* is a good choice and is available at bookstores. It's better than most food counters because it lists the percentage of calories from fat as well as total calories and fat grams. Be honest and accurate when calculating your calories, and when you're done you'll know how many calories you need on an average day to maintain your current weight.

Your goal now is to reduce the calorie level you just calculated by approximately 400 calories through a number of small and relatively easy changes of roughly 35 calories each. (Don't, however, consume fewer than 1,200 calories without medical supervision. If you think you need to consume fewer than 1,200 calories, read Tip 896 for information on finding health-care professionals.) This moderate 400-calorie reduction would take only 10 to 12 days if you were to make a single 35-calorie change each day. If you think a change each day would be too fast, then make one 35-calorie change every other day, or one each week—whatever works best for you. The following is an example of how a 400-calorie reduction list might appear after 12 days:

Small Changes in My Daily Foods

		Calories Reduced
Day 1.	Switch from Cinnamon Toast Crunch to Wheaties	= 21
Day 2.	Cut 1 tablespoon peanut butter at lunch by one-third	= 30
Day 3.	Switch from potato chips to pretzels	= 36
Day 4.	Cut 1 tablespoon margarine on morning toast by one-third	= 33
Day 5.	Switch to reduced-calorie ranch dressing	= 50
Day 6.	Reduce added oil in all dishes by ½ tablespoon	= 60
Day 7.	Stop eating skin on chicken and turkey	= 45
Day 8.	Switch to nonfat American and mozzarella cheese	= 30
Day 9.	No sausage or pepperoni on pizza slice at lunch	= 40
Day 10.	Just taste, don't sample meals in kitchen	= 30
Day 11.	Switch from Campbell's to Hormel minestrone soup	= 26
Day 12.	Switch from lean to extra-lean ground beef	= 18
		TOTAL = 419

Before reducing your calories, be sure to check with your physician to determine if you have any medical problems that require special attention. Once you're ready, start by making the changes you feel are easiest first, and your success is likely to motivate you to continue. You might want to focus first on reducing your consumption of empty calories from sweets and alcohol such as candy bars, doughnuts, soda, beer, or wine. After you've reduced your consumption of these items, you could then move on to everyday fatty foods such as butter, oil, high-fat snacks, sandwich condiments, fast foods, or salad dressings. As you make your reductions, try your best to substitute low-calorie alternatives for your favorite foods, rather than eliminating them altogether. For instance, switch from one tablespoon mayonnaise to one tablespoon mustard or fat-free mayonnaise and you'll save 43 calories. Switch from regular cola to diet cola and save 149 calories for each 12 ounces you drink. Switch from Life cereal to Bran Chex and save 21 calories per serving. Switch from whole to 2-percent milk and save 36 calories per cup. By focusing on substitution rather than elimination, you'll feel much less restricted as you reduce your calorie intake.

With the rapidly growing number of tasty low-calorie foods available today, reducing your calories doesn't have to be a bland and depressing activity. The days of melba toast and Jell-O are over! Read labels of appealing new products, browse your fat and calorie guide, read the Healthy Options Food List in Step 2, the snack list in Tips 61 to 99, and the food chapter (Chapter 8) in Part II of this book for ideas.

If your goal is weight maintenance, then continue through all seven steps of this plan until you stop gaining weight. Once you stop gaining weight, start this 7-Step Plan again by coming back to the Small Changes Approach in Step 1. This will recalculate your calorie and fat intake so that you can start losing weight. If your goal is to lose less than 30 pounds, then continue through all seven steps of this plan until you've lost your weight. If you need to lose more than 30 pounds, then continue through all seven steps of this plan, but once you've lost your first 30 pounds rest and focus on maintaining your weight for at least a month. During this rest period you can consume more calories than when you were losing; just don't consume so many that you start to gain weight. This rest will give your body and mind time to adjust to your new weight and life. After you've rested, perform the Small Changes Approach in Step 1 and all of Step 3 over again before you attempt to lose your next chunk of weight. This will tailor your calorie and fat intake to your new body weight. Continue to lose your weight in this way, losing no more than 30 pounds at a time, until you reach your goal weight.

Step 2.

Maximize Your Satisfaction Through Balance

The true key to satisfaction doesn't lie in quantity, but rather in balanced quality. For your body, balance means satisfaction. The best way to ensure an adequate balance of nutrients at your new calo-

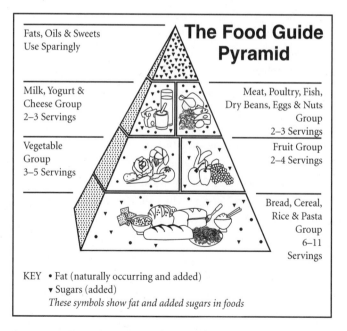

The Food Guide Pyramid

Fats, Oils & Sweets
Use Sparingly

Milk, Yogurt &
Cheese Group
2–3 Servings

Meat, Poultry, Fish,
Dry Beans, Eggs & Nuts
Group
2–3 Servings

Vegetable
Group
3–5 Servings

Fruit Group
2–4 Servings

Bread, Cereal,
Rice & Pasta
Group
6–11
Servings

KEY • Fat (naturally occurring and added)
▾ Sugars (added)
These symbols show fat and added sugars in foods

Source: U.S. Department of Agriculture/U.S. Department of Health and Human Services

rie level is to follow the general guidelines in the Food Guide Pyramid, shown in the diagram. The food-servings checklist and Healthy Options Food List that follow will make using the pyramid easy. Use the pyramid to give structure and balance to your new diet. You can also use the daily menus in Appendixes A and B as a source for planning your meals. If you're pressed for time or not in the mood to cook, you'll find Appendix B especially helpful.

The pyramid is smallest at the top because this uppermost section contains the foods that should be eaten sparingly. The food groups then become a larger and larger part of your diet as you progress toward the bottom of the pyramid.

To make it easy to track your daily servings, I've included a convenient food-servings checklist as part of the monitoring form in Appendix D. It looks like this:

Today's Servings from Food Groups

Milk, Yogurt, Cheese	☐	☐	☐						
Meat, Poultry, etc.	☐	☐	☐						
Fruits	☐	☐	☐	☐					
Vegetables	☐	☐	☐	☐	☐				
Breads, Cereals, etc.	☐	☐	☐	☐	☐	☐	☐	☐	☐

All you have to do is check off your servings as you eat them throughout the day. Don't become too concerned about eating the right number of servings. If you happen to miss a serving one day, just do your best to eat better the next day. Most people find it too difficult to weigh or measure every serving while they're losing weight. Weighing or measuring the foods you eat at the start of your weight-control effort, and as a reminder once or twice a month thereafter, however, can be helpful in developing and maintaining a good visual sense for what constitutes a serving. This is important because most people eat larger servings than they should, according to research at the University of Minnesota. The following guidelines, which are designed for adult men and women, will also help you develop a natural sense for serving sizes.

Bread, Cereal, Rice, and Pasta Group: Eat six to eleven servings per day. Six servings are appropriate for most women; nine servings for most men. Try consuming two servings from this group with each meal (men may want more).

- 1 slice of bread
- ½ bagel, English muffin, or hamburger roll
- 1 ounce ready-to-eat cereal
- ½ cup cooked pasta, rice, or cereal
- 3 or 4 plain crackers

Fruit Group: Eat two to four servings per day. Try consuming at least one fruit serving with each meal.

- 1 whole piece of fresh fruit, or a wedge of fresh melon
- ¾ cup juice
- ½ cup canned, chopped, or cooked fruit
- ¼ cup dried fruit

Vegetable Group: Eat three to five servings per day. Try consuming at least one vegetable serving with lunch and two with supper.

- 1 cup leafy raw vegetables
- ½ cup chopped raw or cooked vegetables
- ¾ cup vegetable juice

Milk, Yogurt, and Cheese Group: Eat two to three servings per day. Pregnant or lactating women, teenagers, and young adults to age 24 should have three servings.

- 1 cup milk or yogurt
- 1½ ounces natural cheese
- 2 ounces processed cheese

Meat, Poultry, Fish, Dry Beans, Eggs, and Nuts Group: Two or three servings per day. Two servings is plenty for most adults. One serving equals two to three ounces of cooked lean meat. A three-ounce serving of either cooked lean beef, poultry, or fish is about the size of the following:

- A deck of playing cards
- An average hamburger
- The palm of your hand

Typical portions of one egg, half a cup of cooked dry beans, or two tablespoons of peanut butter equal one-third of a serving. You can also think of these portions as being equal to one ounce of meat.

The Healthy Options Food List

The following list is designed to give you a quick-reference source you can glance at to plan your balanced meals according to the Food Guide Pyramid. It can be especially helpful if you need a limited number of food choices when first changing your diet. If you think selecting healthy foods from specific lists might help you when you're first starting, then you can eat from just this list and snack from the list of healthy snacks in Tips 61 through 99. Once you become comfortable eating these foods, you can slowly add others. Don't make the mistake, however, of thinking this is a list of "good" foods. There are no good and bad foods, just good and bad eating habits. You don't necessarily have to limit yourself to these choices. Just use this list as a quick-reference guideline. When you're in a hurry, it's easy to forget all of the different kinds of healthy foods that are available. The Healthy Options Food List is organized into the same food groups as the Food Guide Pyramid, with one additional category listing condiments.

Bread, Cereal, Rice, and Pasta Group

BREADS:
Bagel
Bread stick, crisp
Croutons, low-fat
English muffin

French bread
Hard dinner roll
Italian bread
Melba toast
Pancake, low-fat
Pita
Pumpernickel bread
Raisin and other dried-fruit bread

Rye bread
Tortilla, baked
Waffle, low-fat
Whole-grain bread
Zwieback

BREAKFAST CEREALS:
All Bran
Bran Chex
Bran flakes
Cheerios (regular and Honey Nut)
Cream of Rice
Cream of Wheat
Grape Nuts
Kix
Malt-O-Meal
Oatmeal
Puffed wheat
Shredded wheat
Special K
Total
Wheat Chex
Wheaties

CRACKERS AND CHIPS:
Animal crackers, low-fat
Graham crackers, reduced-fat
Keebler Wheatables wheat snack
   crackers
Lay's Baked Original Potato Crisps
Mother's Potato Snaps
Nabisco 5-Grain Harvest Crisps
Nabisco SnackWell's Classic
   Golden Crackers
Oyster crackers
Pretzels

Pringles light chips
Rice cakes
Saltines
Tortilla chips, low-fat or fat-free
   (try Baked Tostitos)
Triscuits, reduced-fat
Wheat Thins, reduced-fat

GRAINS:
Amaranth
Barley
Buckwheat
Corn
Cracked wheat (bulgur)
Millet
Oats
Rice, brown, wild, or white
Rye
Sorghum
Triticale (cross of rye and wheat)
Wheat

PASTAS MADE FROM:
Buckwheat
Corn
Durum wheat
Semolina
Whole wheat

Fruit Group

FRESH FRUIT:
Apricot
Banana
Blackberry
Blueberry
Cantaloupe

Cherry
Currant
Grape
Grapefruit
Honeydew melon
Kiwi
Lemon
Lime
Loganberry
Mandarin orange
Mango
Nectarine
Orange
Papaya
Pear
Persimmon
Pineapple
Plum
Pomegranate
Raspberry
Strawberry
Tangerine
Watermelon

DRIED FRUIT:
Apple
Apricot
Date
Fig
Mango
Peach
Pear
Pineapple
Prune
Raisin

Vegetable Group

Artichoke
Arugula
Asparagus
Beet green
Bell pepper
Broccoli
Brussels sprouts
Butternut squash
Cabbage
Carrot
Cauliflower
Chili pepper
Corn
Cucumber
Dandelion
Kale
Pea pod
Potato
Pumpkin
Romaine lettuce
Spinach
String bean
Tomato
Turnip green
Watercress
Zucchini

Milk, Yogurt, and Cheese Group

Buttermilk, low-fat
Cheeses, low-fat or nonfat
   (no more than 50 calories per
   ounce)
Cottage cheese, nonfat or
   1 percent

Cream cheese, nonfat

Dry milk, nonfat

Evaporated skim milk (some
people enjoy this in coffee)

Frozen yogurt (try Dannon Light
Peach Raspberry Melba)

Ice cream, reduced-fat or fat-free
(try Healthy Choice Rocky Road)

Milk, skim or 1-percent

Sour cream, nonfat

Yogurt, nonfat (no more than
100 calories per cup)

Meat, Poultry, Fish, Dry Beans, Eggs, and Nuts Group

BEANS:

Adzuki beans

Garbanzos (chickpeas)

Kidney beans

Lentils

Lima beans

Navy beans

Peas, green or black-eyed

Pinto beans

Red beans

Refried beans, vegetarian (low-fat
or fat-free)

White beans

EGGS:

Egg substitute

Egg whites

Yolks, no more than four total per
week from all food sources

FISH:

Cod

Flounder

Haddock

Snapper

Sole

Tuna (fresh or packed in water)

OTHER SEAFOOD:

Clams

Crab

Mussels

Oysters

Scallops

Shrimp

LAMB:

Leg chop (lamb steak)

Leg of lamb

Sirloin chop

LUNCHEON MEATS:

Healthy Choice or other low-fat
luncheon meats

PORK:

Ham, very lean (if precooked, at
least "97 percent fat free")

Tenderloin, trimmed

Vegetarian [try Wholesome and
Hearty Foods, Inc.,
Gardensausage, available in the
frozen foods section or call
(800) 636-0109]

POULTRY:

Chicken breast, skinless

Cornish game hen breast, skinless
Turkey bacon
Turkey breast, skinless

RED MEATS:
Eye-of-round, trimmed
Tip round, trimmed
Top round, trimmed
Veal (except ground veal)
Vegetarian [try Wholesome and
  Hearty Foods, Inc.,
  Gardenburger, available in the
  frozen foods section or call
  (800) 636-0109]

Fats and Oils Group

Avocado
Canola oil
Mayonnaise, nonfat
Margarine, for spreading
  (try Fleischmann's Fat-Free
  Low Calorie Spread)
Margarine, for spraying
  (try I Can't Believe It's Not
  Butter! spray)
Olive oil
Peanut butter, reduced-fat or
  substitute (see Tip 293 for
  easy recipe)

Condiments

Applesauce
Barbecue sauce
Bean spread, seasoned nonfat
Capers

Chutney (consists of fruit, spices,
  and herbs)
Cranberries
Cucumber
Extracts and flavorings
Fruit, dried
Fruit butters such as apple
Fruit salad (great on pancakes
  and waffles)
Fruit salsa
Garlic
Horseradish
Hot fudge sauce, fat-free
  (try Wax Orchards flavored
  fudge sauces at gourmet stores)
Jams and jellies
Ketchup
Lemon (fruit or grated peel)
Lime (fruit or grated peel)
Maple-flavored syrup,
  reduced-calorie
Mushrooms
Mustards
Onion
Orange (fruit or grated peel)
Peppers, bell and chili
Pickles
Radishes
Relish
Salad dressing, low-fat or nonfat
  (see Tips 239 to 249 for easy
  recipes)
Salsa
Seafood cocktail sauce
Sauerkraut

Soy sauce

Sprouts

Tabasco

Tamari sauce

Tomato, sun dried (not packed
  in oil) or fresh

Vinegars, traditional and flavored

Worcestershire sauce

Step 3.

Fine-Tune Your Fat Intake

Pick a typical weekday and count the number of fat grams you're consuming at your new calorie level using the form in Appendix D. (Tips for using all of the form will be discussed in Step 4. For now use it to count just fat grams.) After you've done this you'll know how much fat you consume on an average day. Now you have to decide whether you want to maintain or lose weight. Here are your fat intake goals for these two choices:[5]

- To maintain weight, your goal is 25 percent of calories from fat.
- To lose weight, your goal is 20 percent of calories from fat. Once you've reached your goal weight, increase your calories from fat to 25 percent.

In Table 1, My Daily Fat-Gram Allowance, find your new calorie level discussed in Step 1 and then look at the Percent of Calories from Fat column to determine how many fat grams you should be consuming. If you'd like to figure your fat-gram intake on your own, then perform the easy calculation described below the table. Compare the figure from the table, or that you calculated on your own, with the number of fat

---

[5]If you have heart disease, you should consult with your physician and together consider a diet with 10 percent of your calories from fat. A 10-percent fat diet has been proven to reverse heart disease! You might also want to read Dr. Dean Ornish's *Eat More, Weigh Less.*

Table 1

My Daily Fat-Gram Allowance

	Percent of Calories from Fat	
Calorie Level	25%	20%
1,100 calories	31 grams	24 grams
1,200	33	27
1,300	36	29
1,400	39	31
1,500	42	33
1,600	44	36
1,700	47	38
1,800	50	40
1,900	53	42
2,000	56	44
2,100	58	47
2,200	61	49
2,300	64	51
2,400	67	53
2,500	69	56
2,600	72	58
2,700	75	60
2,800	78	62
2,900	81	64
3,000	84	67
3,100	87	69
3,200	90	71
3,300	92	73
3,400	94	76

To determine your daily fat grams for any calorie level, multiply the calorie level by the percentage of fat in your diet, then divide this total by 9. For instance, if you consume 2,000 calories and want your percentage of calories from fat to be 25 percent, then $2,000 \times .25 = 500$. This total is the number of calories contributed by fat in your diet. Divide 500 by 9 (the number of calories in a gram of fat) and you end up with a daily fat allowance of 56 grams.

grams you recorded for an average day. If your fat-gram intake is too low, then you should increase it to the appropriate level. You'll also have to eat fewer complex carbohydrate calories from foods such as bread, potatoes, beans, or pasta to compensate for your increase in fat calories. To figure how many complex carbohydrate calories you need to cut to make room for more fat calories, multiply 9 (the number of calories in a gram of fat) by the number of fat grams you just added. For instance, if you need to raise your fat intake by 3 grams, that's 3 multiplied by 9, or 27 fewer calories from complex carbohydrates you should now eat.

If your fat-gram intake is too high, then lower it through small changes by picking one or two food items, and then focusing on reducing your consumption of just them. If you need to limit your fat intake even more, then once you've controlled these first one or two food items, move on to one or two additional items. Continue to take it one or two items at a time until you've reached your daily fat-gram goal. Once you reach your goal, you'll be able to eat more complex carbohydrate calories from foods such as bread, potatoes, beans, or pasta, since you'll be eating fewer fat calories. To figure how many complex carbohydrate calories you can consume to fill the void created by fewer fat calories, multiply 9 (the number of calories in a gram of fat) by the number of fat grams you just cut. For instance, if you just cut 4 fat grams from your diet, that's 9 multiplied by 4, or 36 additional calories in the form of complex carbohydrates you can now eat.

Tips 222 to 361 focus on practical ways to reduce the fat in your diet. You can use Table 2 as a guide to help you visualize foods that are high in fat. Look it over carefully. You might be surprised to learn, for instance, that whole milk, most fast food, and poultry with skin contain about the same percentage of calories from fat as ice cream!

Table 2

Percentage of Calories from Fat in Some Common Foods

Under 10%	10–25%	25–40%	40–55%	55–70%	Over 70%
Skim milk	1% milk	2% milk	Whole milk	Eggs	Peanut butter
Shrimp	Chicken breast	Dark poultry	Poultry with skin	Tuna in oil	Hot dogs
Scallops		Salmon		Tofu	Bologna
Rice	Turkey breast	Lean pork	Regular ground beef	Sweet breads	Bacon
Egg white	Buttermilk	Lean ground beef	T-bone steak	Yogurt bars	Sausage
Sherbet	Ice milk		Veal	Herring	Spam
Dry beans	Dry cocoa	Soybeans	Granola	Mozzarella	Mayonnaise
Nonfat: milk cheese yogurt	Most seafood	Reduced-fat cheese	Eggnog	Parmesan	Butter
	Low-fat: yogurt cottage cheese	Lamb	Ham	Ricotta	Pepperoni
Fruits		Liver	Rump roast	Romano	Nuts and seeds
Vegetables		Trimmed beef: flank sirloin	Evaporated milk	Provolone	Most cheeses
Hard candy	Trimmed beef: top round eye-of-round tip round		Most fast food: Whopper Big Mac KFC breast fries	Milk chocolate	Margarine
Fruit juice				Fried perch	Nondairy creamer
Special K				Veal	Whipped cream
Wheaties			Ice cream		Ribs
Bran Chex					Pork chops
Malt-O-Meal					Avocado
Cream of Wheat					Coconut
Pasta					Coleslaw
Jell-O					
Berries					
Bread: wheat French mixed grain pita					
Jelly beans					
Sponge cake					

Step 4.

Have a Reality Check Once a Week

Many people consistently underestimate how many calories they eat during the day. In a 1992 study published in the *New England Journal of Medicine*, participants on average underestimated how many calories they ate during a single day by 1,000 calories! They weren't being deceptive. They just appeared to be in a state of denial about how many calories they really consumed. Check in with reality once a week by adding up your calories and fat grams for a typical weekday using the form in Appendix D. Guidelines for actually using the form are also in Appendix D. What follows next are general guidelines that will enhance your overall record keeping:

- Record your food intake immediately so it's as accurate as possible. You may want to carry a pocket-sized notebook or a small tape recorder in which to make your entries throughout the day. You can then transfer these entries to your monitoring form at the end of the day.

- Unto thine own self be true. Don't ever lie in your personal records. Lying to yourself just doesn't make any sense. You're keeping records for yourself and no one else. Be truthful, or you'll only end up hurting yourself in the long run.

- Record everything. Try not to leave out anything you eat or drink. Include the foods you taste during preparation. At first this will be hard, and then when it becomes easier, it will be so easy that you'll find it boring and repetitive. Stick with it, however, and you'll have done much to ensure you'll lose your weight and keep it off.

- As a last resort, try talking out loud. If even using a small notebook or tape recorder once a week sounds too difficult, take a few minutes after dinner to say *out loud* to yourself everything you've eaten during the day. This will help you become more aware of the kind and amount of food you eat. If later you discover you're not losing weight, and you're following the exercise guidelines discussed next, then try written or tape-recorded records.

Step 5.

Build Aerobic Activity into Your Life

Activities that last at least 15 minutes, are continuous, and you can enjoy doing at a comfortable pace are called *aerobic* activities. The fuel mixture your body burns during aerobic activity contains roughly 50 to 60 percent fat. This is significantly more than the 30 to 40 percent fat burned during start-stop activities, which are not aerobic. Consequently, to lose weight as efficiently as possible, you need to participate regularly in one or more aerobic activities. Walking is the overwhelming favorite. Here's a list of aerobic activities from which you can choose. Helpful advice and contact information for major organizations revolving around these activities can be found in Tips 501 to 671. You'll also find a consumer's guide to home-exercise machines in Tips 494 to 500, and a consumer's guide to exercise videos in Tips 539 to 593.

Aerobic dancing (includes Latin, swing, square, and others if
   done continuously)
Back-country skiing or snowboarding
Cross-country skiing (exercise machine or traditional)
Cycling (exercise machine or traditional)
Hiking
Ice skating or speed skating
In-line skating (Rollerblading)
Jogging

Orienteering
Rope jumping (moderate and constant)
Rowing (exercise machine or traditional)
Snowshoeing
Stair climbing (exercise machine or traditional)
Swimming
Walking (exercise machine or traditional)

To lose weight and achieve a moderate level of fitness, you should perform one or more of these aerobic activities at moderate intensity 30 minutes to one hour five to seven days a week, according to the Michigan Health Council. You can achieve this goal in 15-minute blocks or all at once. If you have trouble doing it for 15 minutes, then try doing three sets of 5 minutes each, and gradually work your way up to 15 minutes. Be sure to have fun and progress slowly, so you don't burn out. If you can't do three sets of 5 minutes each, then do just one or two sets of 5 minutes each, and gradually work your way up to three sets of 5 minutes each. Again, your ultimate goal is 30 minutes to one hour five to seven days a week. Start to think of exercise as you do sleeping, working, and eating. Build it into your daily routine. And remember, it's always a good idea to check with your physician before starting any new exercise program.

Once you've reached your goal weight, you can start experimenting with less weekly exercise time. Maybe you'll need to exercise at moderate intensity for only 30 minutes three days a week to maintain your weight. Keep track of how reducing your weekly exercise time affects your mood, self-confidence, calorie and fat-gram intake, and body shape, then experiment to discover what's best for you.

What's moderate intensity? There are two ways to ensure you're burning fat as efficiently as possible by exercising at moderate intensity. The easiest method is called *fitness talk* and will work for any aerobic activity except swimming. The other method uses your pulse and an *aerobic target zone*. You can use either method or a combination of both.

Fitness talk is nothing more than the ability to carry on a conversation while you exercise aerobically. If you find yourself gasping for breath and unable to talk, then you're working out too hard. In other words, you want to work out as hard as you can while carrying on a comfortable conversation. Some highly conditioned people can exercise quite hard and still be able to fitness talk, while others find it difficult to exercise easily and fitness talk. Experiment to discover what works for you, and always go by how you feel. Except for some minor soreness and aches in the first few weeks, your exercise should be painless. Listen to your body and not your mind so that you don't overdo it.

The other method that will ensure you're exercising efficiently uses your pulse and an aerobic target zone. You determine your aerobic target zone by first subtracting your age from 220 to arrive at your maximum heart rate. You then multiply your maximum heart rate by 65 percent (.65) and 80 percent (.80) to determine the boundaries for your aerobic target zone. For instance, if you're 40 years of age, then 220 minus 40 produces a maximum heart rate of 180 beats per minute. This 180 then multiplied by 65 percent equals 117; multiplied by 80 percent equals 144. Consequently in this example your aerobic target zone would be from 117 to 144 beats per minute. If you're a highly trained and healthy athlete, then you can increase the upper limit of your aerobic target zone to 90 percent. You determine your beats per minute by counting heartbeats on the carotid artery in your throat. To do this, gently place your first two fingers next to your Adam's apple on only one side of your throat immediately after you stop exercising. Count your beats for 15 seconds, then multiply this number by 4 to arrive at your beats per minute.

You can use your aerobic target zone to customize your workout based on how you feel and on how much time you have for exercise. For instance, if you feel strong and healthy, you can exercise in the upper range for an intense workout. If you feel weak or tired, you can exercise in the lower range so that you don't stress your body. If you don't have much time, the upper range will give you the best workout in the least time.

This general guideline applies to roughly 60 percent of people. The other 40 percent find their hearts beat too rapidly or too slowly for this rule to help them. If you don't think this rule applies to you, then your best option at this point is to use common sense. Stay in touch with how your body feels. Push yourself so that you feel as if you're getting a good workout, but don't push yourself so hard you feel tired and sore. You may want to try keeping fitness records to track how you feel after your workouts, then adjust the intensity of your workouts according to your records.

Step 6.

Energize Your Day with Little Things

D on't bother trying to add up all the calories you burn each time you exercise. It's not the calories you burn while you exercise that's important. What's really important is that through exercise you're improving your mental outlook and changing your body's chemistry. The sense of well-being, accomplishment, and control over life that exercise gives you is far more important than the number of calories you burn while you're exercising. These psychological benefits are priceless and will enhance not only your weight control, but also your desire to remain active, changing your entire life! What's more, exercise alters your body's chemistry so that it may naturally burn more calories. According to research at the National Institutes of Health metabolism lab in Phoenix, Arizona, lean body tissue is responsible for 80 percent of the calories you burn over a 24-hour period. Consequently, the goal of your exercise should be to make yourself as happy, lean, and muscular as you can be, not to burn X number of calories doing a particular activity.

An easy way to increase your level of physical activity is to find all sorts of little activities you can do throughout your day. It's the total energy (calories) your body spends over a 24-hour period that really counts, which helps to explain why obesity has doubled in America since 1900. All the little things we used to do by hand or foot every day of our lives have decreased dramatically. Energy-saving devices such as electric car windows instead of hand cranks, electric garage-door openers, electric can openers, electric mixers, electric food processors, gas-powered lawn mowers, elevators, escalators, and so forth have all combined to help make us fat. The amount of energy that people used to expend just living day to day even 20 years ago is enormous compared with what we expend today. Consequently you should always be on the lookout for little things you can do to increase your daily activity level. Here are some ideas to get you started:

- Don't send your kids on errands you can do yourself.
- Walk the dog instead of letting him run in the backyard.
- Buy a cordless phone and pace or walk while you talk.
- When you take public transportation, get off several blocks before or after your destination so that you have to walk.
- Walk after dinner instead of watching TV.
- Run and play with your kids instead of watching them.
- Place the trash can in your office in a corner and walk to throw trash away.
- Don't use moving walkways.
- Whenever you run an errand and have extra time, always park far enough away from your destination that you have to walk for five or ten minutes to get there.
- Walk to speak to a colleague, rather than calling him or her on the phone.
- Take your groceries to the car yourself.
- Park several blocks away from your workplace.
- Walk while solving a problem.
- Stand instead of sitting as much as possible.
- Instead of taking the elevator, take the stairs to reach your office.
- Walk down the hall during your coffee break.
- Find a way to walk five minutes during each hour of your day.

Each one of these small acts may not seem like very much. When done daily and added up over time, however, the consequences are enormous. For instance, at 180 pounds you burn about 350 calories an hour when you walk. If you add 2 hours of walking a week, consisting of lots of little walks, that's 104 hours a year. In other words, all those little walks add up to a whopping total-calorie burn of 36,400 calories a year! Since 3,500 calories are stored in each pound of body fat, that means doing all those little extra things could enable you to lose roughly 10 pounds of flab over the course of a single year. This can't be emphasized enough. Every single little thing you do to make yourself more active counts.

Step 7.

Customize and Troubleshoot Using the 1,001 Simple Tips in Part II

You now should be consuming fewer calories in the form of tasty, well-balanced meals, having a reality check once a week, finding little things you can do to be more active, and starting to exercise aerobically at moderate intensity 30 to 60 minutes five to seven days a week. Congratulations! You're leading a healthy lifestyle that will reduce your weight. But you might be thinking to yourself, "Will I be able to continue with this lifestyle?" This is where *1001 Simple Ways to Lose Weight* differs from other weight-control books. Instead of leaving you to grope in the dark on your own with a handful of recipes as other books do, the 1,001 simple tips in Part II of this book will help you customize and troubleshoot your weight-control program. Perhaps you want to add some body-toning exercises to your aerobic routine. Tips 483 to 500 focus on body shaping. Maybe you crave a snack. Tips 61 to 99 contain a listing of tasty low-calorie snacks. What if you wake up and just don't feel motivated? Tips 760 to 792 contain many practical suggestions for getting yourself motivated. What if suddenly you don't feel there's enough time during your day for exercise? Tips 875 to 889 will help you find more time for weight control. Think of Part II as your personal expert advisor, and consult it whenever you have a question or problem.

As you read Part II, keep in mind it's structured so that you can pick and choose the ideas you find appealing. Don't read it from start to finish as if it were a novel. It's designed as a quick-reference guide. If you're already familiar with a tip, or you don't like a tip, then by all means skip it and go on to the next. Your goal is to find tips that work for you. Using the table of contents as your guide, just browse through the pages, jotting down tip numbers for ideas you think will help you achieve your diet and exercise goals. You could also use Part II as a supplement to other approaches that have helped you in the past. Or, if you prefer, you can use Tip 896 to find a health-care professional and use Part II as a supplement to the professional's own approach.

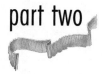

part two

1,001 Simple Ways to Lose Weight

8.

Food Tips[6]

Controlling Mealtime Eating

1. **Drink at least one glass of water before you eat.**

2. **Eat from elegant plates dark in color.** Avoid eating from stoneware, wooden, and brightly colored plates. These stimulate your appetite. If you don't have any dark-colored plates, instead of buying a new set of plates, buy a single setting for yourself either at a garage sale or new.

3. **Eat in rooms with cool colors such as blue or gray.** Avoid eating in rooms with warm hues such as red, orange, or yellow.

4. **Try not to do anything else while you eat, such as reading the newspaper or watching television.**

5. **Don't eat all over the house.** Stay out of the den, bedroom, bathroom, or living room. Make one place in your house your special eating-only place. Don't use it to play board games or cards or to pay bills. Use it just for eating.

6. **Make eating special by dimming the light and setting the table nicely.** Place fresh flowers on the table.

---

[6]It's always a good idea to consult your registered dietitian or physician before changing your diet. If you don't have a professional to turn to for advice, see Tip 896 for information on finding professionals.

7. **Eat with smaller silverware so that you take smaller and more numerous bites.**

8. **Serve food on small plates.** Small plates make moderate servings look like a lot of food.

9. **Eat soup and salad first.** They fill you up and cut down on calorie consumption during your meal.

10. **Chew your food very slowly and savor every bite.**

11. **Put your utensil down between bites.** Try not to have a fork or spoon in your hand if there's food in your mouth.

12. **Try not to feel stressed while eating.** Relax with deep breathing. Hot tea also helps by relaxing both you and your stomach.

13. **Take a tea break.** Put on a pot of water at the start of your meal. When it boils, take time out to rest during your meal with a cup of tea.

14. **Leave the table.** As soon as you feel satisfied place both hands firmly on the table and then push yourself away from the table.

15. **After you're up from the table, leave the house immediately and go for a walk.** When you return you'll feel healthy and more self-confident and so will be much less likely to binge while cleaning the kitchen.

16. **Limit the amount of food you put on the table.** Leave your serving dishes in the kitchen and place only portions on the table. If it's a really creative meal you spent a lot of time on, then try placing your food in an attractive manner on the kitchen counter.

17. **Serve only one portion at a time.** For instance, if you want two pieces of bread make one portion, sit down and eat it, then go and make another portion and sit down and eat it. You may frequently find that you don't eat the second portion because you're no longer hungry after you've finished the first.

18. **Try not to sit around and chat with food still on the table.** Clear the table as soon as everyone is finished.

19. **Have someone else clean up the kitchen.** You made the meal, you bought the groceries, what's unfair about asking your family to put the food away and do the dishes? Clean-up can be a very dangerous time. It's all too easy to stand in the kitchen and mindlessly eat a little more of this item and of that item. Before you know it you've consumed the caloric equivalent of another dinner! Instead, go for a walk while your family cleans up the kitchen. When you return you'll feel great about yourself, refreshed, and ready to spend a fun evening with your family.

20. **Remember the 20-minute rule.** It takes about 20 minutes for your brain to recognize that you're full. The solution is to eat slowly. If you eat too fast, then you'll simply outrace your body's internal controls. Try eating hot soup. You can't eat it fast and it's relaxing, healthy, and satisfying.

21. **Avoid eating for two or three hours before you go to sleep at night.**

22. **Begin your meals with foods high in complex carbohydrates such as beans, whole-grain breads, and pasta.** For instance, eat whole-grain toast first at breakfast. Eat lentil or pea soup before anything else at lunch. Eat pasta, potatoes, rice, or barley before anything else at dinner. By preloading your body with complex carbohydrates first, you'll be less likely to eat fatty foods later.

23. **Start planning your meals.** Planning meals makes life much easier, and yet few people actually do it. You won't believe what a difference just a little planning can make. For starters, try to plan your meals a week in advance. Make an effort to work in one new recipe each week. After you decide what you're having, write out a list of ingredients. Double-check to ensure you have the proper condiments and herbs, such as lemon and dill for salmon, yogurt and parsley for baked potato.

24. **Take it one meal at a time.** The idea of changing how you eat for an entire lifetime is overwhelming indeed. Don't think about the changes you're making in huge, epic terms. Rather, take it one day and one meal at a time and do the best you can each day.

25. **Shift your focus from food to fun during special occasions.** Whether it's a special party at a friend's house or a week on a cruise ship, there's nothing like a special occasion to help you rationalize that you can eat whatever you want. Avoid this by shifting your focus from food to fun. The following two tips will give you some ideas:

26. *Become the game guru for dinner parties.* To ensure the party will be lots of fun and not just idle chitchat around a table filled with food, take an active role in planning. Go to a bookstore and buy several books about games that contain hundreds of games each and the rules to play them. My favorite is Richard Frey's *According to Hoyle.* At your next party, eat, clear away the food, and then play games and chat. This way you'll have a great time that won't center on food.

27. *Plan your vacations.* Before you leave on your next vacation, go to the library and check out books that describe your proposed destination. Use your research to plan activities such as mountain biking through interesting sites, walking through monuments or museums, hiking for a great view, or swimming in a crystal-clear lake. Combining physical activity with sight-seeing is fun, it burns calories, and it's a great way to experience a new place. Of course you can still enjoy eating regional foods. With some planning, however, food won't be the main focus.

28. **Don't focus only on what you can't eat.** Today there are many wonderful light and healthy foods. Don't focus on the few high-fat foods you have to limit. Focus instead on the huge variety of healthy foods you can still enjoy whenever you want such as sweet dates and raisins, seedless grapes that burst in your mouth, bright juicy oranges, seedless watermelon, succulent honeydew, sweet peas,

steamy potatoes, zesty pastas, lean meats, satisfying whole-grain breads, and more.

29. **View healthy food as energy and strength food.** Try not to view foods such as whole-grain breads and pastas, lean meats, veggies, and fruits as bland and boring diet foods. According to research at the University of Alabama, Birmingham, people not only can find low-fat meals as tasty as high-fat meals, but they also can feel full sooner and naturally consume substantially fewer calories. When allowed to consume all the low-fat foods they wanted, participants on average consumed 1,570 calories a day. Shockingly, when allowed to consume all the high-fat foods they wanted, the same participants on average consumed 3,000 calories a day, even though they felt the low-fat and high-fat foods were equally tasty. That's twice the calories! Low-fat foods are without doubt the healthiest and most satisfying choice. Take time to learn how to prepare fast and flavorful low-fat meals and, when eating them, focus on the uplifting feeling these energy and strength foods give you.

Snacking

30. **Store high-calorie foods in opaque containers.** If you can't see the lasagna or cookies inside, then that's one less eating stimulus with which you'll have to cope.

31. **Keep healthy snacks visible and accessible.** Keep enticing bowls of luscious fresh fruit out in the open and take time each night before you go to bed to cut up a bunch of veggies to have as quick snacks for the next day. You can also try carrying a pocketknife and fresh fruit so that you can slice and eat your fruit whenever you want.

32. **Buy foods that you have to prepare.** Food that is ready to eat is so accessible that you're very likely to overeat. You don't want to have ready-to-eat foods handy that you can just stuff into your mouth on impulse. Try to have only ingredients from your menu plan around the house. This way you'll have to work for your meals.

33. **Avoid buying foods for later.** Avoid buying foods "to use later." Out of reach is often out of mind. Try to keep all excess food out of the house. As you're probably well aware, all too often that food you bought for later ends up in your mouth just a few hours after dinner.

34. **Limit your exposure to fatty, sugary food advertising.** How many times have you been peacefully watching television when suddenly you're hit with an advertisement for chocolate ice cream loaded with calories, or for pizza packed with salt and fat? Your VCR can help you avoid this. Tape the shows you want to watch, and then while watching them fast-forward through the advertisements.

35. **Give away what you don't eat.** Many people love to cook. It's a creative outlet for them that reduces daily stress. Of course the problem is that the more they cook, the better they become, and the harder it is for them not to eat their creations. To avoid eating everything you make, give your extra food away immediately. Try baking treats for neighbors with kids who don't have time to bake, for a shut-in or an elderly person, or for a food kitchen or shelter for homeless people. The key here is to get a list of people who love and need your cooking.

36. **Ride out the craving.** Cravings start slowly, build steadily to a peak, and then subside. Think of your craving as a wave that slowly builds and then subsides, and try to wait it out.

37. **Brush, floss, and rinse after you eat.** This idea is popular because it works. Brush and then floss your teeth after every meal and when you feel like bingeing. When your mouth feels clean and fresh you're less likely to stuff food into it. You can also use a fluoride rinse after dinner. You shouldn't eat for several hours after rinsing with fluoride.

38. **Keep food out of the automobile.** Driving and eating resembles eating and watching TV. You can consume 3,000 calories and not even know it! Don't eat and drive. If you must eat while driving, snack on veggies or dried fruit and sip water.

39. **Avoid skipping meals.** It's common for people to skip meals thinking they're doing themselves a big favor by cutting back on calories. This usually doesn't work. Not only does it make you very susceptible to bingeing on fatty and sugary foods later in the day, but it also slows your metabolism.

40. **Avoid skipping breakfast in particular.** It's revealing that one factor common to overweight people is that they seldom eat breakfast. This can be for many reasons ranging from a simple lack of time, or not feeling hungry, to thinking they're saving themselves calories by skipping breakfast. Breakfast is an essential part of your diet and crucial for limiting your total daily calories. Eating breakfast, especially one high in fiber, helps control your calorie intake for the rest of the day by preventing you from finding yourself famished later. Experiment with the ideas in Tips 41 through 46 and put a stop to your breakfast skipping:

41. *Take a few minutes to plan your breakfast the night before.* This way you'll have your breakfast ready to eat when you wake up. Your breakfast can either be a breakfast-to-go such as fruit and low-fat cheese, or one that will require some additional preparation in the morning such as a fresh-blended frozen fruit drink.

42. *Focus on simple breakfasts when you're in a hurry.* Breakfast doesn't have to be complicated. Just eat foods such as fresh fruit, whole-grain toast, English muffins, instant breakfast mixes, yogurt, bagels, or ready-to-eat breakfast cereals. If you opt for the ready-to-eat cereal, choose one that is low in salt and sugar and high in fiber.

43. *Try waking up 10 to 15 minutes earlier to make more time for breakfast.* You probably won't miss the sleep, and this will give you plenty of time to consume cereal, fruit, and a glass of juice.

44. *If you're not hungry, drink some natural fruit juice and take something to eat on the way to work such as a bagel or English muffin.*

45. *List five to seven low-fat breakfasts on 3" × 5" cards and refer to them when you're rushed in the morning.* This tactic makes your breakfasts easier to prepare and adds variety to your breakfasts.

46. *Involve others.* Get your family or friends to eat breakfast with you and to help with the planning and preparation. It's usually very nice to eat with other people, and they can help to ensure you don't skip breakfast.

47. **Try eating on a strict schedule.** Some people can control their eating better if they maintain a strict schedule. They eat three or four meals a day at the same time every day. Because they've trained their bodies to become hungry at certain times of the day, they reduce between-meal snacking.

48. **Try eating with no schedule at all.** Some people control their weight better by grazing throughout the entire day and never really eating an official meal at all. They just eat a number of small and nutritious meals and snacks throughout the course of their day. This keeps their blood sugar stable and so makes them less susceptible to mood swings. They also never become ravenous and end up in a situation where they're likely to binge.

49. **Create an eating-alternatives list to cut between-meal snacks.** For instance, your list might include playing a musical instrument, kissing somebody, reading a romantic book, planning a vacation, visiting a fitness-conscious friend, reading this book, taking a drive, shopping for flowers, working on a hobby, and so forth. Keep the list visible so that you always have something to do when you shouldn't be eating.

50. **Avoid oily chips and crackers.** These are almost always high in fat. Usually when the label says light, the company means the chip or cracker is low in sodium. Always opt for baked and not fried, and try the crunchy substitutes listed in Tips 51 through 58:

51. *Hot-air popcorn*

52. *Baked tortilla chips*

53. *Matzos*

54. *Fat-free crackers*

55. *Peppers*

56. *Carrots*

57. *Broccoli*

58. *Cauliflower*

59. **Limit candy bars.** This may seem obvious, but candy bars are so compact and tasty that they often appear more innocent than they actually are. A single two-ounce candy bar contains close to 300 calories, can make you moody, and can actually stimulate your appetite. It's okay to enjoy them once in a while; just don't get in the habit of eating them often to satisfy yourself between meals.

60. **Store snacks in serving sizes.** If you find yourself confronted with an entire package of snacks, try using sandwich bags to package the snacks separately into serving sizes. Your family may think it's weird, but this will force you to notice exactly how much you're eating so that you'll be less likely to overeat.

61. **Substitute tasty low-calorie snacks for binge foods.** Next time you arrive home from work late, stressed, starving, and with no dinner in sight, instead of bingeing before you can get a nutritious meal in you, try one of the binge busters listed in Tips 62 through 99. Each binge buster is under 150 calories. I've listed a number of sweet treats because it's often better to have sweet treats in limited amounts than it is to deny them completely. Sugary binge busters should be followed, however, by a nutritious meal. Consuming sugar on its own can make you moody and hungry:

62. *One cup Swiss Miss hot cocoa mix.* Warms you up and fills your mouth with the taste of chocolate. Even the original flavors have only 110 calories per one-cup serving. Try these, or the new low-calorie flavors with only 20 calories per one-cup serving.

63. *About 20 Teddy Grahams.* These little teddy bear cookies are tasty and fun to eat. If you're in a panic situation, eat your 20 or so and then get rid of the rest.

64. *One large York Peppermint Pattie.* Great when you're hungry, tired, or at a store shopping and need something to keep you from pigging out before dinner.

65. *Fifteen jelly beans.* If you have never tried gourmet jelly beans, then do yourself a favor and try them (JellyBelly brand are best). Each one seems to explode with a burst of satisfaction when you pop it into your mouth.

66. *One slice Entenmann's Fat-Free Fudge Brownie.* Whoopee!

67. *Pizza pizzazz.* Take four low-salt whole-grain crackers and top each with a tablespoon of low-fat pizza sauce or tomato sauce. On top of that put a tablespoon of sliced or chopped veggies such as broccoli, mushrooms, or peppers. On top of that put a one-eighth-ounce slice of nonfat mozzarella cheese. Broil until the cheese melts and serve them hot. All four add up to only 112 calories!

68. *Frozen grapes.* This classic binge buster consists of taking high-quality red seedless grapes and freezing them. They taste like sour balls when you eat them.

69. *Brussels sprouts with almonds and blue cheese.* This makes four servings, and one is only 127 calories. Take three pints of fresh brussels sprouts, steam or microwave them, then drain thoroughly. In a food processor or mixing bowl, mix two tablespoons of blue cheese with one tablespoon of margarine and one tablespoon of finely chopped almonds. Add this mixture to the brussels sprouts and enjoy.

70. *Spiced popcorn.* Using a one-quart saucepan, simmer on low heat one minced garlic clove in one tablespoon of olive oil for one minute. Now stir in one-half teaspoon of dried basil and one-half teaspoon of dried parsley. Stir for 30 seconds, then drizzle over eight cups of popped corn. Sprinkle two tablespoons of grated Parmesan cheese over the top and it's done. This makes four servings.

71. *Cauliflower or broccoli Italian style.* Take a medium head of cauliflower or broccoli and break it apart into florets. Heat your wok or large skillet to a medium-high temperature for about 30 seconds. Now add one tablespoon of white wine and one-half teaspoon of olive oil, then heat for an additional 20 seconds. Reduce heat, add four cloves of finely minced garlic, then stir constantly until it just starts to brown. Add cauliflower or broccoli and stir for two to three minutes. Add one-quarter teaspoon pepper, two tablespoons red wine vinegar, two tablespoons water, and one tablespoon chives. Cover and cook over low heat for 10 minutes more. This makes four servings at 56 calories per serving.

72. *Toasted chickpeas.* This is rapidly becoming a classic because it tastes terrific. Heat one-half cup of drained garbanzos on a tray for five minutes in a toaster oven and sprinkle a favorite seasoning such as Mrs. Dash over the top.

73. *Two Keebler Elfin Delights Chocolate Sandwich Cookies with Fudge Creme.*

74. *Simple apple salad.* Combine one-half cup of raisins, one-third cup of chopped walnuts, and six cups of chopped, unpeeled red delicious apples in a bowl and gently toss together. In a separate bowl combine two tablespoons of honey with one-half cup of vanilla low-fat yogurt and stir well. Add this honey/yogurt mixture to the apple mixture and gently toss to coat. Chill covered for about one hour. This will produce eight ¾-cup servings at 134 calories per serving.

75. *Two Mrs. T's Pierogies.* These are low-fat pasta pockets packed with oniony cheese/potato filling.

76. *Sweet fruit or melon with ice.* Grab your blender, take some sweet fruit or melon such as nectarine, orange, grapefruit, peach, strawberry, or watermelon, and blend together with ice to desired consistency. This is especially good during the summer. Just be sure your fruit or melon is ripe and sweet.

77. *One Häagen Dazs Piña Colada Frozen Yogurt Bar.* A coconut and pineapple miracle.

78. *Weight Watchers Chocolate Mousse.* Only 35 calories per bar and super taste.

79. *One-half cup Häagen Dazs sorbet of choice.*

80. *Four frozen bonbons.* They take longer to eat when frozen.

81. *Four waffle creme cookies.* Light and sweet.

82. *Three-quarters cup Jell-O.* Festive and visually appealing.

83. *One-half cup Healthy Choice Chocolate Fudge Mousse or Rocky Road ice cream.* As good as the "real thing."

84. *One half-inch slice banana bread.* Try it warm without butter or margarine.

85. *Three tablespoons candy corn.* Be sure to have a toothbrush handy.

86. *Icy fruit salad.* Combine three-quarters cup each of sliced ripe banana, grapefruit sections, red seedless grapes, cubed fresh pineapple, and unsweetened pineapple juice in a large bowl. Add one-eighth cup of water and one-eighth cup of undiluted and thawed frozen orange juice concentrate. Mix together, then pour into a 13″ × 9″ × 2″ baking dish. Freeze covered for about eight hours or until firm. To serve, let stand at room temperature for one hour and serve slightly thawed. Makes four servings with 125 calories per serving.

87. *Cinnamon sweet potato.* Pierce a sweet potato with a fork, pop it into the microwave for five to seven minutes, sprinkle it with cinnamon, and enjoy.

88. *Three regular-sized chocolate chip cookies.* It's hard not to eat the whole carton in a panic situation. You'll be better off if you can buy them three at a time.

89. *Two or three fat-free SnackWell's cookies.* The fat-free have only 50 calories per serving compared with 110 calories per serving in the "reduced-fat" version. These taste super.

90. *One ounce of three-ring pretzels.*

91. *Fruit smoothy.* Blend one-half of a frozen banana, one-half cup of frozen peaches, or other frozen fruit of choice with one cup non-fat skim milk.

92. *Frozen yogurt.* One-half cup frozen hard-packed or soft-serve yogurt with two teaspoons topping of choice such as fresh fruit, berries, or sprinkles.

93. *Two fat-free fig bars.*

94. *One ounce of fat-free cheese puffs.*

95. *One cup cinnamon applesauce.* One cup unsweetened applesauce sprinkled with cinnamon.

96. *New Zealand fruit mix.* Mix together one-half of a sliced kiwi, one-half cup pineapple chunks, and one-half of a banana.

97. *One frozen fruit-juice bar.*

98. *Orange-strawberry shake.* Blend together one-half of a six-ounce can of slightly thawed orange juice concentrate, eight ounces whole frozen strawberries (without sugar), one-half cup nonfat vanilla yogurt, and one cup skim milk.

99. *Piña colada treat.* Blend together one small banana, two tablespoons nonfat dry milk powder, one-half cup nonfat plain yogurt, one tablespoon fresh lime juice, one-half cup drained pineapple chunks, two teaspoons sugar, and one-eighth teaspoon coconut extract.

Nutrition

100. Remember the difference between bad fats and not-as-bad fats.
Try to make the small amount of fat you do consume *unsaturated* fat so that you reduce your chances of clogging your arteries. The best unsaturated oils for keeping your blood cholesterol healthy and reducing your risk of heart disease are canola oil and olive oil. Severely restrict *saturated* fats such as butter or lard that come primarily from animal sources. Consume too much saturated fat, and your arteries could look like the one in the illustration below. Do all of your cooking with olive or canola oils and, when necessary, use a tub or liquid margarine that's nonhydrogenated. My favorites are I Can't Believe It's Not Butter! spray and Fleischmann's Fat-Free Low Calorie Spread.

Blocked Artery

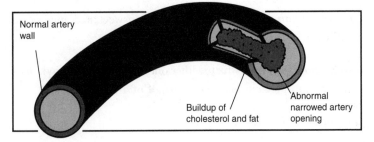

Normal artery wall

Buildup of cholesterol and fat

Abnormal narrowed artery opening

101. Pay attention to calories and fat grams for the entire day. For instance, if you happen to arrive to work late starving and stuff a cream-filled doughnut into your mouth, don't get depressed. It's okay. You still have your entire day ahead of you. Cut back on your calories and fat grams at lunch and dinner, and your fat intake for the day as a whole will be just fine. If it's not, then do your best to cut back some more the next day as well. Everyone slips up at one point or another. Just tell yourself to relax and then try to do better at your next meal.

102. **Consume enough fiber.** There are two kinds of fiber. One is called *water-soluble* and has been shown to reduce cholesterol levels. Good sources of water-soluble fiber are barley, oatmeal, rice, legumes (beans and peas), and carrots. The other is called *water-insoluble*. Water-insoluble fiber may reduce your risk for colon cancer and may help control your appetite by adding fat-free bulk to your diet. Good sources of water-insoluble fiber are fruits, vegetables, whole grains, and legumes. Follow the guidelines in the Food Guide Pyramid and you'll receive enough fiber in your diet.

103. **Reduce your sodium intake.** To significantly lower your sodium intake, limit your consumption of processed foods. According to the March 1994 issue of *Nutrition Action Healthletter*, 15 percent of the sodium in our diets comes from the shaker, 10 percent is found naturally in food, and more than 75 percent comes from processed foods! In particular, processed cheeses, cured foods, and canned foods such as soups, vegetables, or broth can be high in sodium. To reduce your sodium intake, eat more fresh and home-made foods and opt for low-sodium versions of processed foods. Don't, however, get carried away and cut out all the sodium in your diet. Too little sodium can cause muscle cramping, dizziness, weakness, confusion, and palpitations. The recommended daily allowance for adults is 1,100 to 3,300 milligrams of sodium, which is three to eight grams of salt (one teaspoon is about five grams).

104. **Understand the power of a calorie.** Voluminous research has made it clear that calories most definitely do count. For instance, let's say you simply add one-eighth teaspoon of mayonnaise extra to your sandwich at lunch every day. That translates into just 10 puny calories extra a day. No big deal, right? *Wrong!* Over a single year those 10 extra calories could lob an entire pound of fat onto your body. Over 10 years you could gain 10 pounds of flab. Now imagine that you eat 100 calories more per day than you need. This could mean a weight gain of 10 pounds over the course of a single year!

105. **Calculate calories and fat grams based on your true portion sizes (what you really eat).** Don't assume the "per serving" information on the label tells what you're actually eating. Try the following tips designed to help you avoid two classic weight-control traps:

106. *Check your portion sizes.* Many serving sizes listed on food labels are unrealistically small. Consequently, by the time you've finished a normal serving you've eaten more fat grams and calories than you probably realize. Multiply the number of servings you'll actually eat by the calories and fat grams per serving on the label in order to understand how many calories and fat grams you're really eating.

107. *Limit your consumption of drinks containing sugar or alcohol.* Because drinks come in liquid form and you can guzzle 16 ounces in seconds, it's sometimes easy to forget they too can be loaded with calories. This is especially true of alcoholic drinks. A piña colada, for example, contains roughly 450 calories! Drink lots of water instead.

108. **Drink water in small sips to quench cravings.** Most people know they should drink six to eight glasses of water each day. Many people, however, don't know that it's not so much the amount you drink, but rather *how often* you drink that's the key to quenching food cravings. According to research at Boston's New England Deaconess Hospital, small three- to four-ounce quantities of water sipped often throughout the day will satisfy your cravings better than eight ounces all at one time. Also, remember that your goal with sipping is to satisfy thirst and reduce food cravings, but not to stimulate your taste buds. Consequently sip water, not tea, soda, coffee, or juice.

109. **Eat pasta, whole-grain breads, and other complex carbohydrates.** There are two groups of carbohydrates. One group is called *simple sugars*—found in foods such as syrups, soda, candy, and many processed foods. The other group is called *complex carbohy-*

drates—found in beans, whole grains, and vegetables. Many people still mistakenly think that eating pasta, whole-grain breads, and other foods high in complex carbohydrates will make them fat. The fact is, you actually burn more calories in the process of using food high in complex carbohydrates than you do using food high in fat. This is a major reason why the most servings per day in the Food Guide Pyramid consist of foods high in complex carbohydrates. Foods such as pastas and whole-grain breads don't in themselves make you fat, but high-calorie toppings certainly do. Try putting spicy sauces, tomatoes, peppers, and herbs on your pasta to give it a zestful flavor without fat. Sprouted wheat bread is naturally sweet. Or try adding dried fruit such as chopped dried cranberries, sour cherries, blueberries, or apricots to your favoriate bread recipe for a wonderful sweet flavor.

110. **Don't do the high-protein diet.** This is a scam. The weight loss on a high-protein diet is very impressive during the first few weeks, but this is due to water loss. Worse still, some weight-loss programs that are mainly protein can lead to a potentially serious condition called acidosis. Symptoms can include malaise, heart arrhythmias, weakness, and headache. Forget diets that emphasize one nutrient such as protein. Balance and moderation are the only two things you need to remember for good nutrition during weight control. Even people who eat small portions of protein-rich foods generally get more protein than they need. As long as you eat regular balanced meals and adhere to the Food Guide Pyramid, you'll receive enough protein in your diet.

111. **Limit or avoid alcohol.** Alcohol is second only to fat in calories and stimulates your appetite.

112. **Avoid severely restrictive diets and stop dieting insanity.** Never go on a diet that severely restricts what you eat or drink, like the grapefruit or cabbage diet. These diets are scams and, in many cases, dangerously unhealthy. Going on a restrictive diet is a lot like trying to hold your breath for the rest of your life. You just

can't do it. After a while the body will take control and force you to breathe or eat even if you don't want to. Worse still, just as your body was designed to gasp for air after restricted breathing, it will crave a large number of calories after restrictive dieting to make up for caloric deprivation. The result is the characteristic post-diet binge.

113. **Realize nondairy doesn't always mean low fat.** Some nondairy items such as Ice Bean, Rice Dream, or Tofutti sound really healthy, and you'd think they'd make a good substitute for ice cream. The fact is, however, they too are usually high in fat. They don't have any cholesterol because they contain soybeans, sugar, water, and oil, but they can have lots of fat. Always try to buy frozen desserts with three or less grams of fat per one-half cup.

114. **Understand there are no vitamins that promote weight loss or provide energy.** There's no evidence anywhere that proves any vitamin, or any combination of vitamins, will help you lose weight. Don't fall victim to vitamin advertising that says or implies they will. The truth is, nutrition experts generally believe that most people in the developed world who eat a balanced diet don't need to take any vitamin supplements at all. In addition, none of the 14 known vitamins will give you more energy. Some vitamins help the body use energy from fats, carbohydrates, and proteins, but these are easily supplied by healthy food. Focus on eating healthy balanced meals using the Food Guide Pyramid.

115. **Limit consumption of caffeine.** Without caffeine you may get off to a slower start in the morning, but you'll have much more energy over the course of the entire day. With caffeine you'll start out fast and then crash suddenly, making you moody and more likely to binge. A more consistent and natural caffeine-free energy pattern may prove more beneficial to you over the course of an entire day, as opposed to an artificial pattern of caffeine highs and lows.

Meal Planning and Kitchen Tips

116. **Develop strategies to avoid sampling when you prepare food.**
Use the following tips to get started:

117. *Sip water or herbal tea.*

118. *Chew sugarless gum.*

119. *Have your spouse in the kitchen.*

120. *Don't eat out of an original container.* The large size will make
you think you're eating less than you actually are.

121. *Prepare your meals immediately after you finish eating.* For
instance, after you finish eating dinner, make low-fat lasagna and
refrigerate it for your next lunch or dinner.

122. *Prepare fatty dishes immediately after breakfast and then store
them out of sight until needed, if you must make them at all.* Most
people find fatty foods less appealing during the morning hours.

123. **View meats and cheeses as condiments.** Try to stop thinking of
meats and cheeses, which are high in fat, as a large part of your
main courses. Instead think of them as condiments that sometimes may be needed to add flavor to your low-fat entrees.

124. **Make certain that you really are hungry before you eat.** Try these
tips to see if you really are physically hungry:

125. *Take a short walk.* If you return even hungrier than before, then
you probably do need to eat.

126. *Ask yourself on a scale of 0 to 10, with 0 being empty, 5 being
comfortable, and 10 stuffed, how hungry are you?* Eat when you
feel you're at about 2, and then continue eating only until you
reach 5.

127. *Drink a large glass of water or a cup of hot tea.* Wait 10 minutes
and see if you're still hungry.

128. *Just wait 20 minutes and see if you're still hungry.*

129. **Understand that occasionally high fat can be better than low fat.** Sometimes you may consume fewer calories and fat grams if you eat a small portion of a high-fat food instead of a large portion of a low-fat food. For instance, if you don't find the low-fat brownies you're eating very satisfying, you may be eating so many of them that you're consuming more total calories and fat grams than if you just ate a small portion of traditional high-fat brownie. ·

130. **Try not to food shop on an empty stomach or with a lot of money.** Doughnuts and cookies are extremely tempting when you enter a grocery store starving. Eat before shopping. As extra protection against buying high-fat foods, don't shop with a credit card, ATM card, or checkbook. Take only enough cash for what you have on your list. If you do happen to find yourself in a grocery store starving and loaded with cash, then walk only the outside aisles where you'll find mostly vegetables, breads, fruits, or low-fat dairy products. Chewing sugarless gum while you shop also helps.

131. **Make your kitchen an efficient low-fat kitchen.** Low-fat cooking can be much easier with the proper equipment. Tips 132 through 152 list equipment you may want to consider acquiring:

132. *Make frozen ice milk, yogurt, fruit ices, and sorbet in an ice cream maker.*

133. *Use an egg separator to remove the yolks from eggs.*

134. *Try a clay cooker.* A dampened clay pot will allow your meat to simmer slowly in its own juices without adding any fat or liquid.

135. *Coddle eggs in an egg coddler.* These are easier to prepare than poached eggs.

136. *Steam foods such as dried beans, peas, or chicken in a short time using a pressure cooker.*

137. *Simmer your fish in herbs and veggies in a fish poacher instead of frying.*

138. *Use a food processor to grate, julienne, cut, and do all sorts of things that your blender can't.*

139. *Check portion sizes on a kitchen scale.*

140. *Use quality Teflon or stainless steel nonstick pans.* Don't skimp here. Also, use a high-grade plastic spatula that won't scratch or melt. Wooden spoons work best for stirring.

141. *Get a ridged-bottom cast-iron skillet.* The ridge will keep fat away from your food, and the skillet is good for grilling.

142. *Place a meat and poultry rack in your pans to allow the fat to drain away from meat.*

143. *Use a gravy separator to separate fat from liquid in soups and sauces.*

144. *Use a skimmer to skim fat from sauces and soups.*

145. *Try a wok.* This is a deep-sided pan that will allow you to stir fry using almost no fat.

146. *Use a strainer to rinse all of the fresh fruits and veggies you're eating now.*

147. *Use a slow cooker to save time when preparing one-pot meals and healthy homemade soups.*

148. *Try a mortar and pestle for grinding your herbs before you add them.* Do this even to herbs you buy ground up. It will make a big difference in the flavor.

149. *Use a double boiler to prepare sauces and reheat leftovers.*

150. *Experiment with a yogurt maker.* This is a cost-effective way to have tasty, healthy yogurt on demand.

151. *Keep your knives handy and sharp to slice and dice your fresh foods.*

152. *Get a spaghetti measurer.* Have you ever cooked too much spaghetti and then overeaten so that you didn't waste any? You can prevent this from happening with this simple and cheap device.

153. **Try listing your danger foods.** Before you start your next and final weight-control effort, you may want to set aside some time to identify your personal danger foods. Use your list as a guide to reduce your consumption of them.

154. **Experiment with fresh and spicy foods to enhance your food's flavor and texture.** Try the following tips:

155. *Grind your own spices.* Grind pepper and nutmeg at the table to make your light dishes as flavorful as possible.

156. *Freeze garlic to keep it fresh.* When you're ready to use a clove, peel it, then thaw it.

157. *Use a spice chart to help you spice up dishes in a hurry.* Table 3 gives you a place to start. You can list your foods either alphabetically or by frequency of use.

158. *Buy a fridge thermometer and keep your fridge on the cold side at between 32 and 38 degrees.* This will keep your foods fresh without harming produce or freezing liquids.

159. *Place paper towels or dry sponges across the bottom of your vegetable bin to reduce moisture and keep your fruits and veggies fresher longer.*

160. *Start with the freshest foods possible.* Don't try to save money by using old limp fruits and veggies. Without fat for flavor, the food itself will have to taste good on its own. Droopy lettuce and soggy celery just won't work.

Table 3

Spices, Herbs, and Accompaniments

Poultry, Fish, and Meat

- Poultry: Thyme, poultry seasoning, sage, lemon juice, fresh mushrooms, fruit chutney, bell peppers, parsley, marjoram, paprika.
- Fish: Bell peppers, lemon juice, bay leaf, curry powder, dry mustard powder, paprika, marjoram, fresh mushrooms, pineapple salsa.
- Beef: Fresh mushrooms, bell peppers, nutmeg, bay leaf, onion, garlic, pepper, dry mustard powder, thyme, marjoram.
- Pork: Sage, garlic, onion, apple, applesauce.

Vegetables

- Potatoes: Parsley, bay leaf, bell peppers, mace, onion, pepper, paprika, caraway seeds, basil.
- Rice: Bell peppers, fresh mushrooms, chives, onion, saffron, pimiento.
- Tomatoes: Garlic, oregano, onion, basil, marjoram, pepper, bell peppers.
- Peas: Fresh mushrooms, savory, onion, bell peppers, parsley, mint.
- Green beans: Lemon juice, dill, nutmeg, marjoram, pimiento.
- Corn: Fresh tomato, bell peppers, pimiento.
- Cucumbers: Vinegar, dill, garlic, chives, basil.
- Squash: Nutmeg, brown sugar, ginger, cinnamon, mace, onion.

161. *Take care of your lettuce.* How many times have you gone to the fridge, tired, hungry, wanting to eat a healthy salad, only to find the lettuce is wilted and rotten? Every single time you arrive home from the grocery store spin your lettuce dry, and then store it in an airtight container with a paper towel to keep it fresh for as long as possible.

162. *To prevent brown spots after you cut into the core of a head of iceberg lettuce, instead of cutting, hit the core sharply against a counter top and twist to remove.*

163. *Try storing lettuce and celery in a paper bag with the outer leaves attached.*

164. *Wrap green bananas and tomatoes in a wet dish towel, then place in a paper sack to ripen.*

165. *If your bananas are very ripe, freeze them for a tasty treat.*

166. *Perforated plastic bags work well to ripen fruits.* The bag retains the ethylene gas fruits produce to help them ripen, and the holes allow for some air movement.

167. *Toss a quart or two of freshly cut fruit with the juice of half a lemon to prevent the fruit from becoming dark.*

168. *To get more juice from your lemons, store them whole in a closed jar of water in the refrigerator.*

169. *If your bread becomes dry, you can bring it back to life by wrapping it in a damp towel and placing it in the refrigerator for 24 hours.*

170. *Place a rib of celery in the bread bag to keep bread fresher longer.*

171. *Wrap crackers tightly and store in the fridge to keep them crisp even in humid weather.*

172. *When you cook corn, don't add salt to the water—it makes the corn tough.*

173. *Do you want to peel a bunch of potatoes in advance but are afraid they'll turn black or spoil before you use them?* Add a few drops of vinegar to cold water, cover your peeled spuds with it, and refrigerate, and they'll last three to four days.

174. *Rebake leftover baked potatoes by dipping them in water for five seconds and then baking them for about 20 minutes at 350 degrees.*

175. *Rinse frozen vegetables with boiling-hot water before preparing them to eliminate the frozen water in which they came.*

176. *"Old maids" can be reduced in your popcorn by storing it in the freezer and then popping without thawing, or by running ice-cold water over the kernels before you pop them.*

177. **Don't let your meals become bland and boring.** Enliven your meals by experimenting with the following tips:

178. *Enjoy a variety of colors, textures, and kinds of food at each meal.* Plan your meals so that they contain at least three different kinds of food (e.g., bread, fruit, poultry), served at three different temperatures (e.g., warm, cold, hot), and containing three different colors (e.g., brown, orange, white). This sensual variety will make your meals more satisfying.

179. *Get together with your friends once a week to share recipes, then pick your light recipe of the week and test-prepare it together.*

180. *Subscribe to light cooking magazines such as* Cooking Light *or* Eating Well.

181. *Go to your public library and read low-fat cookbooks to find recipes you'll enjoy preparing and eating.*

182. *Take a light cooking course with a friend.*

183. *Plan your meals in advance and test at least one new meal on your family each week.*

184. *Develop an experimental, "I'll try anything" attitude.* Don't be shy or you may miss some great recipes.

185. *Hold friendly cooking competitions with your friends.* See who can find and prepare the tastiest low-fat dishes.

Dining Out

186. **Take fresh veggies to social functions.** Take a plate full of veggies and a low-fat dip to parties or gatherings you attend. This way you know you'll have something healthy, crunchy, and low-fat to

munch on while you chat with others. Most everyone will be glad to have some healthy things to eat, and veggies work the best. They're high in fiber, so they fill you up, and their crunchy texture is very satisfying to chew. Fruit is too perishable and sticky on your fingers.

187. **Plan ahead what foods to choose at fairs, exhibitions, sports events, and amusement parks.** Beware of popcorn popped in palm oil and enjoy the snacks listed in Tips 188 to 194:

188. *Lemonade*

189. *Soft pretzels with mustard*

190. *Cinnamon candied apples*

191. *Sweet corn on the cob*

192. *Nonfat frozen yogurt*

193. *Snow cones*

194. *Frozen bananas*

195. **Plan ahead to eat healthy when you fly.** Tips 196 to 202 will help you control your calorie and fat consumption when flying:

196. *Do yourself a big favor and skip airplane nuts.* The salt makes you thirsty and bloated, and the nuts derive roughly 80 percent of their calories from fat.

197. *Try relaxing with several deep slow breaths instead of drinking alcohol when you're stressed.*

198. *Call ahead and reserve a special meal for yourself when you make your plane reservations.* This doesn't cost extra and requires only 24-hour notice. You might find the seafood platter a consistently tasty and healthy choice.

199. *Request that the high-fat processed dessert be left off your tray.*

200. *Drink a glass of water every hour you're in flight.*

201. *Go with the cold cereal and fruit for breakfast.* Pass up the high-fat sausage and eggs.

202. *Carefully check your itinerary to ensure you're going to get food when you need it.* The airplane and airport are the worst places to be when you're hungry. You're almost always guaranteed a very expensive, poor-tasting, and high-fat meal if you're forced to eat in these places.

203. **Eat healthy even at not-so-healthy restaurants.** Many people have to eat out a lot because of work. This often constitutes an enormous weight-control challenge. Use Tips 204 through 219 to help you plan your strategy:

204. *Buy a low-fat guide to fast-food restaurants.* Every bookstore carries them. They're a fat-saving quick reference when you're in too much of a hurry to visit a sit-down restaurant.

205. *Tell the waiter, "Please either steam or microwave my veggies."*

206. *Always get your butter on the side with items such as potatoes or toast.*

207. *Skip the high-fat appetizers, and, instead, ask for mineral water with a twist of lime or lemon and a salad or veggie plate with dressing on the side.* Keep in mind that most appetizers are purposely high in salt and fat to tease your appetite.

208. *Have the bread basket brought out with the meal, and ask for whole-grain bread.* This way you won't eat two baskets of bread while you're waiting for your meal.

209. *Avoid creamed soups like the plague!*

210. *Keep in mind that "au gratin" means the dish has a cheese sauce, "sauté" usually translates into butter added, and "tempura" equals batter-fried.*

211. *Try low-fat yogurt on your potato instead of butter or sour cream.*

212. *Ask if they can broil your main dish instead of frying it.*

213. *Try to select dishes listed as garden fresh, poached, dry broiled, roasted, or steamed.*

214. *Order your gravy, sauces, and dressings served on the side to ensure your food doesn't arrive swimming in high-fat toppings.*

215. *Instead of pouring dressing over the top of your salad, try dipping your fork into dressing on the side first, and then picking up some salad.*

216. *Choose a baked potato over french fries.*

217. *Eat authentic ethnic foods.* Americanized versions of traditionally healthy Asian and Mexican foods, for instance, are often high in fat and sodium.

218. *To deal with the large portions you often receive at a restaurant, try putting one spoonful in your mouth and the next at the back of your plate or on another plate.* Do this for each bite you take.

219. *Conduct a dry run when confronted with a buffet.* Before you put plate in hand, walk the length of the buffet and decide which healthy foods you'll eat. After you've finished your dry run, go through the buffet with your plate and select only the foods you chose during your dry run.

220. **Avoid "all you can eat" signs.** What happens when you're surrounded by tons of wonderful food at a restaurant and money is no object? It's very hard not to overeat during an all-you-can-eat. Do your best to avoid them.

221. **Avoid the restaurant atmosphere of overeating.** The major problem with eating out is the atmosphere for overeating prevalent at restaurants. There are too many high-fat dishes and desserts that always tempt you. At home you have to buy and then prepare your food. In a restaurant you just order and wham, one super cheesecake ready to stuff in your mouth! Eat at home, keep fatty foods

out of your house, and you'll be more likely to stick with eating moderate healthy meals and snacks.

Cooking and Recipes

222. **Use fat-cutting preparation methods to substantially reduce the amount of fat in your dishes.** Tips 223 through 361 were all kitchen tested and chosen for their simplicity and effectiveness.

Salads, Dressings, and Dips

223. **Use healthy alternatives to bacon bits and cheese chunks on your salads.** To make up for their flavor, try the sprouts listed here, keeping in mind that it's very easy to grow your own in the kitchen:

224. *Peanut sprouts*

225. *Mustard sprouts*

226. *Mung bean sprouts*

227. *Alfalfa sprouts*

228. *Sunflower sprouts*

229. *Radish sprouts*

230. *Fenugreek sprouts*

231. **In addition to sprouts, use the following foods to add flavor to your salad without adding fat:**

232. *Green peppercorns*

233. *Small ears of baby corn*

234. *Minced dill pickle*

235. *Small cocktail onions*

236. *Exotic mushrooms*

237. *Pickled ginger*

238. *Roasted red bell peppers.* To roast, broil them for 20 minutes, or until the skins blister, turning them every 5 minutes. Steam under a tight lid for an additional 15 minutes, peel, seed, and slice.

239. **Experiment with the following flavored vinegars to boost the taste of your dressings:**

240. *Balsamic vinegar*

241. *Tarragon vinegar*

242. *Raspberry vinegar*

243. *Red wine vinegar*

244. *Cider vinegar*

245. **Try to become accustomed to using oil and vinegar salad dressing with approximately a one-to-one ratio of vinegar to oil.** Most traditional oil and vinegar dressings call for twice as much oil as they do vinegar. Soon you won't believe you ever ate such oily salads. Once you're accustomed to a one-to-one ratio, try reducing your oil even more by spraying it on your salad with a spray bottle. This will lightly coat your salad so that the spices will stick, which is the purpose of the oil in the first place. If you don't want to make your own dressings, then invest in a number of low-fat brands to find the one you think tastes best.

246. **Try a creamy low-fat dressing.** A simple creamy low-fat dressing with only three grams of fat and 30 calories per serving (tablespoon), this standard light dressing is a real winner:

Creamy Light Dressing

> 2 tablespoons balsamic vinegar
> 4 tablespoons plain nonfat yogurt
> 1 tablespoon extra-virgin olive oil
> ¼ teaspoon salt

¼ teaspoon finely minced garlic

2 teaspoons minced basil, chives, fresh parsley, or mint

In a bowl, whisk ingredients together until smooth. You can store this in the fridge for several days covered. Whisk again just before serving.

Makes 6 1-tablespoon servings with 27 calories and 2.4 grams fat each.

247. In most creamy dressings containing mayonnaise, usually you can substitute nonfat or soy yogurt, nonfat or soy sour cream, or nonfat buttermilk for the mayo.

248. For a quick Thousand Island dressing, whisk together a half teaspoon of fresh lemon juice and a half-cup of nonfat yogurt. Now fold in two tablespoons of tomato paste and add minced sweet pickles, celery, garlic, and shallots to taste.

249. For a quick ranch dressing, mix one-quarter cup buttermilk with one teaspoon each of Dijon mustard, minced chives, garlic, and parsley.

250. Rub garlic in your wooden salad bowl for a wonderful garlic flavor.

251. Make your salads filling by tossing in kidney beans, chickpeas, brown lentils, or pasta.

252. Mashed tofu is high in protein, relatively low in fat when compared with many animal products, cholesterol free, and a good recipe substitute for cottage and ricotta cheese. Be sure, however, to taste the final product. Tofu has a mild flavor; therefore you'll probably want to add more seasoning when using it as a substitute. Tofu dip can be used as a substitute for mayonnaise, on sandwiches, and in dressings. It keeps well covered in the fridge for about five days. Here's a standard and tasty tofu dip recipe you can try:

Tasty Tofu Dip

  ¼ teaspoon salt
  ¾ teaspoon white pepper
  2 tablespoons lemon juice
  6 ounces soft tofu

SEASONINGS

Finely chopped pickle
Onion powder
Garlic powder

Puree all ingredients until creamy and then adjust your seasonings.

Makes about 7 ounces of dip totaling 104 calories and 4.6 grams fat.

253. Perhaps the tastiest and easiest dip of all is plain nonfat or soy yogurt seasoned with your favorite seasoning.

254. Another excellent dip is leftover soup. Try dipping unbuttered toast or bread in warm leftover soup.

Soups, Sauces, and Toppings

255. Use these foods and ideas to thicken soups without a lot of fat:

256. *Cornstarch*

257. *Farina*

258. *Long cooking over low heat*

259. *Flour*

260. *A diced cooked potato in any blended soup*

261. *A small amount of tofu pureed with water*

262. To reduce the fat in natural meat renderings, try this: Save the renderings in the bottom of a broiling pan. After cooking, defat the meat juice by placing it in a clear heat-proof container and submerging it in ice water up to the level of the juices. This will cause the fat to rise and thicken so you can skim it off.

263. Use the technique in Tip 262 with your soups, stews, and sauces to eliminate that last bit of extra fat.

264. **Ramen noodles are a quick and easy meal.** Just make sure you buy baked and not fried noodles (check the fat content).

265. **Try black bean soup, one of the easiest and best-tasting light soups.** For a super-fast meal, add one-half cup black bean flakes (they're sold in bulk) to a cup of hot water, season with balsamic vinegar or spicy harissa, and steep covered for 10 minutes.

266. **To create a quick minestrone soup base, mix V-8 with tomato juice in equal amounts.**

267. **Next time you make a soup with meat, try using half the meat the recipe calls for.** Slice the meat you do use into small pieces, and then substitute veggies, beans, or pasta for the other half of the meat. You can also experiment with the meat substitutes listed in Tips 268 through 274:

268. *Potatoes*

269. *Cauliflower*

270. *Lentils*

271. *Small shaped pastas*

272. *Garbanzo beans*

273. *Black beans*

274. *Kidney beans*

275. **When oil is absolutely necessary for seasoning foods, use walnut oil, sesame oil, or extra-virgin olive oil.** These oils have strong concentrated flavors so that you can use less of them.

276. **Use foods with highly concentrated flavors instead of butter, margarine, cheese, or cream.** Flavor-packed foods such as garlic, mushrooms, basil, onions, tomatoes, leeks, or fresh parsley fill sauces with flavor without relying on high-fat dairy foods.

277. **Try Butter Buds Butter Flavored Mix.** This is available at your local supermarket and will give you a buttery taste without any fat.

278. **Use the intense color of paprika or crushed saffron threads to make your soups and sauces seem rich.**

279. **Choose cocktail sauce over tartar sauce.** It is much lower in fat.

280. **Use vegetable puree as a sauce instead of an oil-based one.** Puree veggies in the water in which you cooked them, then season and salt to taste.

281. **Try the following to thicken your gravies without much fat.** Most people prefer to substitute one tablespoon of thickener for every two tablespoons of butter called for in the recipe:

282. *Kudzu*

283. *Pureed beans*

284. *Cornstarch*

285. *Arrowroot*

286. **Instead of cheese, use crushed cereal flakes or bread crumbs to top a casserole, pizza, or anything else traditionally topped with cheese.**

287. **Remember that Parmesan is a cheese like any other and is full of fat.** Don't be misled by the fact you sprinkle instead of slice it.

Beans and Bread

288. **Cook a pot of raw beans on the weekend so that you'll have beans handy throughout the week.** Raw beans do take some time to cook, but they more than make up for the extra time in flavor. Prepare them by first rinsing and then soaking overnight. To cook, discard the soaking water and cook with fresh water two to three times the volume of the beans. You can also freeze soaked beans in small serving-size bags to have handy during the week.

289. **Substitute lentils if you're too busy to prepare beans.** Rinse the lentils with cold water, pick out any discolored pieces, and drain in a colander. Cook green and brown lentils about 15 to 20 minutes on the stove. Cook orange lentils 5 to 10 minutes.

290. **Try black bean burritos.** With a zesty salsa, tomatoes, lettuce, mushrooms, and cucumbers, all wrapped up in a whole-wheat tortilla, these are always a winner. Spread beans and salsa on the rolled-up tortilla and heat in the oven until the tortilla is crisp. Serve hot.

291. **Use sage in bean or split pea soup to provide the flavor of ham.**

292. **Heat peanut butter, honey, maple syrup, margarine, and other food items to make them spread more easily so that you can use less of them.**

293. **Try this peanut butter substitute.** Take one tablespoon of peanut butter and mix it with one-quarter cup rinsed, drained, and mashed Great Northern beans. This is good with jelly in sandwiches, plain, or with celery. I personally don't like it on crackers. It has four grams of fat and 70 calories in two tablespoons.

294. **If you can't make your own bread, take time to find the very best bread bakery in your area.** Quality breads are full of flavor and require no topping when eaten warm.

295. **Make corn bread.** It's sweet and tasty and easy to make.

296. **Spread your toast with jelly instead of butter.** A teaspoon of jelly or jam has no fat and only 16 calories.

297. **Try leftover soup on your toast for lunch.**

298. **Heat up a can of vegetarian baked beans to top your toast.** You'll have a wonderful lunch in minutes.

299. **Next time you make a yeast-bread at home, try leaving out the fat.** It probably doesn't really need it.

300. **Don't be fooled into thinking that all muffins are a low-fat choice for breakfast.** Always make sure you're eating low-fat muffins or English muffins. You'll get the same satisfaction with a fraction of the fat.

301. **Eat bagels often.** They come in an exciting variety of flavors and are naturally low in fat, are filling, and when heated don't require any topping.

Grains and Pastas

302. **Test a wide variety of grains to give body to your meals without high-fat meats and cheeses.** You may tire of just using wheat, oats, and rice in your dishes. In particular, try the following grains:

303. *Barley is terrific by itself as a side dish, for breakfast, or in soups, stews, and casseroles.*

304. *You'll be surprised at how fluffy and light millet is.*

305. *Kasha has kept the Russians alive through their long winters for centuries.* It's known here in the United States as buckwheat.

306. **Cook grains in fruit juice to add flavor and moisture.** Try a mixture containing half water and half apple juice.

307. **Prepare dishes using boxed grains to save time.** In America boxed dishes such as quick couscous, lentil pilaf, barley pilaf, and rice pilaf are sold for use as side dishes. They also make wonderful main dishes, however, and are so easy to prepare that they are great for camping and hiking food.

308. **Use exciting rice that doesn't cry out for sauce as plain rice does.** Try aromatic strains such as pecan, basmati, Wehani, or Texmati. These smell like buttery popcorn or roasting nuts and satisfy you all on their own.

309. **Steam corn tortillas instead of frying.** Wrap them in aluminum foil and bake for about 10 minutes in an oven at 375 degrees until flexible and hot. This process is called steam baking.

310. It's not necessary to add oil to boiling pasta to prevent sticking if you use enough water. Use four quarts of water for each pound of pasta. Also, avoid breaking pasta into smaller pieces. This releases starch, making your pasta much stickier.

311. Lighten up lasagna by substituting crumbled tofu for ricotta cheese or by making vegetable lasagna.

312. Lighten up your tuna-noodle casserole. Make it with margarine, skim milk, a few shavings of cheese, and a bit of flour (for thickening) rather than with whole milk and a fat-laden can of creamy condensed soup. Take it to work and microwave it. It's a nice change from sandwiches, and it will stay with you until dinner.

313. For a quick pasta primavera, toss a bag of frozen mixed veggies into your boiling pasta at the end. Drain, spray with a light coating of olive oil, and then dust with Parmesan cheese.

314. Avoid egg noodles. Instead, look for the words "durum wheat" and "semolina" to ensure you're purchasing plain pasta.

Veggies

315. Save your veggie broth in an ice tray. Veggie broth is loaded with vitamins and great to sauté food in and to use in soups, stews, and casseroles. Freeze it in an ice-cube tray and you'll have a quick source of broth in convenient and ready-to-use portions.

316. Sauté in the oven. Coat a nonstick pan with nonstick cooking spray and place your vegetables inside. Place in oven preheated to 400 to 425 degrees and remove when softened.

317. Instead of sautéing vegetables to be used in soups in oil and butter, steam them in a little soup liquid or cook them along with everything else in the soup itself.

318. If you can find no alternative to oil when you sauté, then experiment with using as little as possible. Use one-half to one teaspoon of oil per serving.

319. Add brightly colored veggies to your dishes to make them more visually satisfying.

320. Try a cucumber sandwich. Soak your sliced cucumbers in red wine vinegar and then place them on pieces of thinly sliced bread for a quick and tasty meal.

321. Put moisture into your sandwiches with "wet" veggies such as tomatoes or cucumbers instead of relying on fats for moisture.

322. Experiment with the following toppings to liven up your baked potatoes:

323. *Light soy sauce*

324. *Garlic and basil pasta sauce*

325. *Plain nonfat yogurt*

326. *Tamari sauce*

327. *Oversteamed and mashed cauliflower and broccoli*

328. *Salsa*

329. *Stir-fried vegetables*

330. Try a high-quality baking potato. Slice it in half lengthwise and season with one bay leaf, add salt and pepper to taste, wrap in foil, and bake at 425 degrees for about 40 minutes or until tender. Top with a choice from Tips 323 through 329, or from Tips 331 through 337.

331. *Barbecue sauce*

332. *Oregano*

333. *Ratatouille*

334. *Worcestershire sauce*

335. *Leftover soup*

336. *Grated nonfat cheese such as mozzarella*

337. *Mustard diluted with some mashed tofu*

338. **Enjoy mashed potatoes without milk or butter.** First steam the potatoes and use a hand masher to mash them slightly. While mashing, use enough vegetable water or plain water to create the desired consistency. Whip with an electric beater and season with Mrs. Dash or Hungarian paprika.

339. **Don't fry frozen hash-browns.** First read the label to make sure they aren't made with oil. Next spray a nonstick skillet with nonstick cooking spray and brown over medium heat for about 12 minutes.

340. **Eat white potatoes with golden skin and you'll need less, if any, butter or cheese.** Varieties such as Yukon Gold, Yellow Finnish, or Yellow Rose are naturally rich and flavorful.

Meats

341. **For stuffing, use defatted chicken broth instead of butter or margarine.** Add mushrooms, celery, even raisins for more flavor. Also, don't cook your stuffing inside the bird. Stuffing placed inside the bird acts as a fat-absorbing sponge. Cook it separately and add fat-free chicken or turkey stock as needed.

342. **Instead of using high-fat gravies, marinate poultry and meat in a fruit-based marinade and serve chutney or cranberry relish on the side.** These taste fabulous and don't add any fat.

343. **Poach boned chicken pieces and firm-fleshed fish.** This process maintains flavor and requires very little time. Herbs and vegetables recommended in nonpoaching chicken and fish recipes can be added to the poaching liquid—usually in reduced amounts—for flavor.

344. **Try this exceptionally easy and tasty chicken recipe.** It's great if you love fried chicken but are afraid to eat it because it's high in fat.

San Diego Oven-Fried Chicken

1 cup crushed corn flakes
1 teaspoon garlic powder
1 teaspoon paprika
1 teaspoon thyme
4 skinless chicken breast pieces
½ cup skim buttermilk
1 tablespoon plus 1 teaspoon canola oil

Preheat oven to 350 degrees. Combine crushed corn flakes with garlic powder, paprika, and thyme, then spread over a piece of wax paper. Dip chicken breast pieces in buttermilk, then dredge in corn flake mixture. Arrange chicken in a baking dish and drizzle canola oil evenly over the top. Bake for 30 minutes, turn pieces over, then bake 15 to 20 minutes more, until cooked through.

Makes 4 servings with 363 calories and 10.45 grams fat each.

345. **Avoid chicken wings.** Even though they're often considered white meat, they have more fat than the drumstick!

346. **Always purchase canned fish such as tuna packed in water rather than oil.**

347. **Try cooking fish in parchment paper to retain flavor without adding any fat.** Top fish with herbs, garlic, lemon, onion, or red bell pepper, before wrapping in the parchment.

348. **Soak fish in vinegar and water before cooking for a sweet and tender taste.**

349. **Get rid of the frozen taste of frozen fish by thawing it in milk.**

350. **Replace some of the ground beef in spaghetti sauce, meat loaf, and tacos with lower-fat ground turkey.** If you ask your butcher to grind up the turkey for you without the skin, you'll end up with

even less fat than you might find in prepackaged ground turkey. Don't buy poultry if the label just says "chicken" or "turkey." Look for labels that list "breast meat." About half the fat in chicken or turkey is found in the skin.

351. **When buying red meat, keep in mind the leanest cut is top round, followed by eye, bottom, and tip.** Talk to the people in the meat department of your grocery store. You'll find them helpful when you have questions about which cuts are leanest.

352. **Brown meats using a broiler and the fat will drip away from the meat and into the lower broiler pan.**

353. **Substitute mashed potatoes or rice for some of the meat in your meat loaf.** Also drain off the liquid fat after it cooks, and you'll have substantially reduced the fat in your meat loaf.

354. **Try pita-to-go for a meaty lunch when you're in a hurry.** Stuff a whole-wheat pita with turkey, chicken, tuna, or lean ham and top with veggies of your choice such as broccoli, cauliflower, alfalfa sprouts, butter lettuce, tomatoes, or onions. Finish it with vinaigrette dressing (recipe follows). Complement your pita-to-go with a piece of fresh fruit.

Vinaigrette Dressing

2 tablespoons water
3 tablespoons vinegar
1 teaspoon Dijon mustard
1 tablespoon extra-virgin olive oil
Salt and pepper to taste

In a bowl, whisk ingredients together until smooth.

Makes 6 1-tablespoon servings with 22 calories and 2.35 grams fat each.

355. **Use mustard, fruit, or a vegetable-based chutney to flavor sandwiches made with turkey, chicken, or ham.**

Treats[7]

356. **Whip a can of evaporated skim milk instead of heavy cream.** This will work if the milk, beaters, and glass bowl are cold and free of grease. One cup will yield about five cups of whipped topping. Add a little sweetener or vanilla extract for flavor and then chill.

357. **Cut the fat in most traditional treat recipes by one-third and you probably won't affect the flavor.**

358. **The country's finest light cooks replace up to half of the oil called for in many treat recipes with applesauce measure for measure.** For instance, you could substitute one-third cup of applesauce for one-third cup of butter in your brownies.

359. **To replace body lost with discarded yolks in your light treat recipes, you can try mixing in a dollop of low-fat cottage cheese.**

360. **Eliminate completely or halve the nuts called for in the recipe.**

361. **Use meringue whenever possible.** It's naturally low in fat.

Favorite Light Recipes

362. **Try these all-time favorite simple light recipes.** Here's a list of kitchen-tested light recipes that are both tasty and easy to prepare. The recipes follow the alphabetized index and are in tips 363 through 417.

Alphabetized Index

[7]For an extensive list of tasty low-calorie treats, see Tips 62 through 99.

368. Carrot-Sweet Muffins
369. Cheese and Apple Sourdough Muffins
370. Chive and Pepper Scallops
371. Classic Western Omelette
372. Crispy-Light Scallops in a Flash
373. Decadent Double-Chocolate Goody
374. Easiest Light Microwave Lasagna Ever
375. Easy Baked Herbed Halibut
376. Easy Popcorn Caramel Brittle
377. Energizing Fruit Slush
378. Exciting Mashed Potatoes
379. Fabulous Italian Figs
380. Fast and Flavorful Chicken Salad
381. Favorite Buttermilk Dressing
382. Favorite Butterscotch Cookies
383. Greatest Grapefruit Caesar Salad in the Land
384. Honey Salad
385. Honeydew-Heaven Slush
386. Jamaican Pineapple Treat
387. Leek/Cucumber Salad
388. Light and Tasty Lorraine
389. Light Herb Dip
390. Light Pound Cake
391. *Almond Pound Cake*
392. *Butter Rum Pound Cake*
393. *Butter-Flavored Pound Cake*
394. *Coconut Pound Cake*
395. *Lemon Pound Cake*
396. Manhattan Grilled Sandwich
397. No-Mayo Potato Salad
398. Orange-Basil Salmon Steaks
399. Outstanding Chicken Club
400. Oven Onion Rings
401. Perfect Fruit Punch
402. Pizzazz Corn Bread

403. Quick and Tasty Cauliflower Meal
404. Salad Scrumptious Pizza
405. Sensational Sesame Chicken
406. Sesame-Healthy Granola
407. Shrimp with Tomato Vinaigrette
408. Snappy Mexican Snapper
409. State of the Art Chicken Chili
410. Superb Microwave Sauce "Hollandaise"
411. Superb Sweet Chicken
412. Super-Easy Chinese Chicken
413. Ultra-Fast Breakfast
414. Vanilla-Cherry Soda
415. World's Best Light Cucumber Dip
416. Yogurt-Pudding Chocolate Sponge Cake
417. Your Best Russian Dressing

363. *Almond Cantaloupe Dessert*

¼ cantaloupe, cubed
4 fresh figs, chopped
2 mandarin oranges, peeled and sectioned
1 bunch seedless grapes
¼ cup chopped toasted almonds
1 cup lowfat vanilla yogurt

1. Arrange fruit in a bowl.

2. Sprinkle with toasted almonds and top with lowfat vanilla yogurt.

Makes 1 serving with 250 calories and 1.4 grams fat.

364. *Baby Salad with Smoked Salmon*

1 head baby romaine
2 heads baby red-leaf lettuce
2 heads baby Bibb lettuce
2 heads baby endive

2 heads baby radicchio

½ bunch fresh dill

1 sprig thyme

2 bunches chervil leaves

1 teaspoon chopped parsley

¼ cup rice wine vinegar

½ cup water

2 tablespoons lemon juice

1½ tablespoons olive oil

¼ teaspoon chopped shallots

½ teaspoon freshly ground pepper

¼ teaspoon salt

1 teaspoon Dijon mustard

8 ounces smoked salmon, chopped

2 cups cooked white beans

12 Ak-Mak crackers, crumbled

1. Remove lettuce cores and discard. Wash leaves and gently pat dry. Pick herbs from stems and chop. Toss greens in a large bowl.

2. Place rice vinegar and all remaining ingredients except salmon, beans, and crackers in a screw-top container and shake well. Toss liquid with salad to coat and place on plates. Sprinkle salmon, beans, and crackers over top.

Makes 6 servings with 175 calories and 5.8 grams fat each.

365. *Barbecued Fruit Kabob*

½ teaspoon ground cinnamon

½ teaspoon amaretto liqueur

¼ cup maple syrup

2 tablespoons brown sugar

8 eight-inch wooden skewers

4 kiwis, peeled and quartered

4 bananas, cut into 16 one-inch slices

16 one-inch cubes watermelon
16 one-inch cubes fresh pineapple

1. Heat coals to medium-hot. In a bowl mix cinnamon, amaretto, maple syrup, and brown sugar and set aside. Soak skewers in water for several minutes.

2. Skewer, in order, kiwi, banana, watermelon, and pineapple cubes until each skewer is filled. Brush with syrup mixture and save remaining syrup for marinade. Coat grill with cooking spray and grill fruit, turning after 3 minutes, for a total of 6 minutes. Remove and drizzle with marinade.

Makes 8 servings with 98 calories and 4 grams fat each.

366. Broccoli and Pasta

1 tablespoon olive oil
1 medium onion, chopped
1 orange or yellow bell pepper, sliced
2 cloves garlic, minced
Florets from one large stalk broccoli
1 cup water
6 black olives, chopped
1 tablespoon fresh minced oregano
1 tablespoon currants
1 tablespoon fresh minced parsley
⅛ tablespoon freshly ground black pepper
1 pound cooked pasta
Red pepper flakes

1. In a large nonstick frying pan, heat olive oil over medium heat. Add onion, bell pepper, and garlic.

2. Sauté, stirring, until garlic and onion are golden but not brown (5 to 7 minutes). Add broccoli, water, olives, oregano, currants, parsley, and black pepper, then simmer for 10 minutes.

3. Mix this with cooked pasta and sprinkle with red pepper flakes. Serve while hot.

Makes 6 servings with 299 calories and 2.4 grams fat each.

367. *Caribbean Black Beans*

2 tablespoons chopped and seeded tomato
2 tablespoons chopped green bell pepper
2 tablespoons chopped onion
1½ teaspoons seeded and chopped mild chili pepper
Freshly ground black papper
½ teaspoon olive oil
4 ounces canned black beans, drained and rinsed
⅓ cup water
½ ounce boiled ham, diced
1 cup cooked long-grain rice, warm

1. In shallow one-quart microwavable casserole dish, mix tomato, bell pepper, onion, chili pepper, black pepper, and oil. Toss to coat. Microwave on high until onion is soft.

2. Divide beans in half and mash one-half. Add mashed half to whole-bean half and stir in water, ham, and onion/pepper mixture. Cover and microwave for 7 minutes on high stirring briefly every 2 minutes. Serve over warm rice.

Makes 1 serving with 326 calories and 6.4 grams fat.

368. *Carrot-Sweet Muffins*

¾ cup raisins
1 cup plus 2 tablespoons whole wheat flour
1 cup plus 2 tablespoons all-purpose flour
¼ cup plus 2 tablespoons packed light brown sugar
¼ teaspoon salt
1¼ teaspoons baking powder
½ cup egg substitute

¼ cup melted margarine

1 cup skim milk

1. Preheat oven to 375 degrees and coat twelve 2¾-inch muffin cups with nonstick cooking spray. In a large bowl, stir together raisins, flours, brown sugar, salt, and baking powder.

2. Stir together remaining ingredients and then mix into dry ingredients with a fork until just combined. Spoon batter into cups and bake until toothpick comes out clean, 20 to 25 minutes.

Makes 12 servings with 184 calories and 4 grams fat each.

369. *Cheese and Apple Sourdough Muffins*

3 tablespoons finely chopped purple onion

½ cup low-fat cottage cheese

1 small red delicious apple

2 sourdough English muffins, split and toasted

¼ cup shredded cheddar or crumbled blue cheese

1. Stir together onion and cottage cheese in a small bowl. On each muffin half spread 2½ tablespoons cottage cheese mixture.

2. Core apple and slice crosswise into four ¼-inch rings. Top each muffin with an apple ring. Sprinkle cheese over top, place on baking sheet, and broil 3 inches from heat for 1 to 2 minutes or until cheese melts (watch closely).

Makes 2 servings with 304 calories and 6.2 grams fat each.

370. *Chive and Pepper Scallops*

1 tablespoon reduced-calorie margarine

½ tablespoon olive oil

3 tablespoons chopped fresh chives

2 dried hot chili peppers (optional)
¾ pound fresh scallops
½ red bell pepper
Pinch ground cloves
2 cups cooked wild rice

1. In a skillet, heat margarine and olive oil, then add chives and chili peppers (optional) and sauté for 30 seconds. Add scallops and sauté 2 minutes, or just long enough to heat through.

2. Thinly slice red pepper. Stir red pepper and cloves into scallop mixture.

3. Cook another 30 seconds and serve over rice.

Makes 4 servings with 186 calories and 4 grams fat each.

371. *Classic Western Omelette*

¼ cup finely diced onion
2 tablespoons finely diced red bell pepper
2 tablespoons finely diced green bell pepper
3 ounces cooked potato, diced
1 ounce turkey ham, diced fine
¾ ounce low-fat cheddar cheese, shredded
Dash black pepper
2 teaspoons margarine
¾ cup frozen egg substitute, thawed
¼ cup alfalfa sprouts
1 cherry tomato, halved

1. Cook onion and bell peppers over medium-high heat in a 10-inch nonstick skillet coated with nonstick cooking spray, stirring frequently. Cook about 2 minutes or until onion is soft. Add potato and turkey ham and continue stirring for about 1 minute or until potato is heated through. Remove

from heat and stir in cheese and black pepper. Move to plate, cover with another plate to keep warm, and set aside.

2. Wipe skillet with a paper towel. Melt margarine in skillet and add egg substitute. Cook and stir over medium heat for 30 seconds. Continue to cook without stirring 1½ minutes, until egg substitute is set.

3. Spoon potato mixture into center of omelette, fold omelette in half, and serve garnished with sprouts and tomato halves.

Makes 2 servings with 172 calories and 7 grams fat each.

372. Crispy-Light Scallops in a Flash

3 tablespoons low-fat buttermilk
15 ounces sea scallops, quartered
⅓ cup plus 2 teaspoons seasoned dried bread crumbs
½ teaspoon ground thyme

1. Combine buttermilk and scallops in a medium mixing bowl and marinate at room temperature 15 minutes.

2. Coat a baking sheet with nonstick spray and preheat oven to 500 degrees. Combine bread crumbs and thyme in a small mixing bowl. Dredge scallops in crumbs and place on baking sheet. Bake 5 minutes, carefully turning scallops over until browned on all sides.

Makes 4 servings with 139 calories and 1 gram fat each.

373. Decadent Double-Chocolate Goody

1 envelope instant reduced-calorie chocolate pudding mix
2 cups skim milk
½ cup frozen dairy whipped topping, thawed
1 tablespoon chocolate syrup
1 ounce toasted almonds, chopped
2 maraschino cherries, halved

1. Make pudding according to package directions using 2 cups skim milk. Spoon a quarter of the pudding into each of four 6-ounce dessert dishes.

2. In a small bowl stir to combine whipped topping and syrup. Spread a quarter of the mixture over each pudding portion.

3. Sprinkle a quarter of the almonds over each dessert, and top off with a cherry half. Refrigerate covered for at least 45 minutes.

Makes 4 servings with 155 calories and 6 grams fat each.

374. *Easiest Light Microwave Lasagna Ever*

½ pound lean ground beef (optional)
½ cup water
1 32-ounce jar meatless marinara or spaghetti sauce
1 egg
1½ cups nonfat ricotta cheese
¼ teaspoon each minced garlic, black pepper, basil, and oregano
8 uncooked lasagna noodles
8 ounces low-fat mozzarella cheese, shredded
2 tablespoons reduced-fat Parmesan cheese

1. In a large glass bowl, crumble beef and microwave 2 to 3 minutes on high, or until beef is brown. Drain off fat and stir in water and marinara sauce.

2. Combine egg, ricotta, garlic, pepper, basil, and oregano.

3. Spoon ½ cup of marinara into bottom of 8″ × 12″ microwave pan. Add a layer of four noodles, a layer of half of the mozzarella, a layer of ricotta mix, another layer of marinara, the remaining noodles, the remaining mozzarella, the remaining ricotta mix, and the remaining marinara.

4. Microwave on high for 8 minutes and then on medium-low for 30 to 32 minutes. Let stand 15 minutes. Serve topped with Parmesan.

Makes 9 servings with 287 calories and 6.4 grams fat each.

375. *Easy Baked Herbed Halibut*

4 5-ounce fresh halibut fillets
Juice from ½ large lemon
Dash freshly ground pepper
Dash crushed oregano
Dash crushed basil
1 8-ounce can salt-free tomato sauce
½ cup chopped celery
2 ripe plum tomatoes, chopped
1 small onion, chopped
1 green bell pepper, chopped
6 fresh mushrooms, sliced

1. Preheat oven to 375 degrees. Sprinkle fillets on both sides with lemon juice, pepper, oregano, and basil. Let stand 15 minutes.

2. In the bottom of a shallow baking dish pour a small amount of tomato sauce. Lay fish on sauce, place in upper third of oven, and bake for 10 minutes.

3. On top of fish place celery, tomatoes, onion, green pepper, and mushrooms. Pour remaining tomato sauce over top and bake for an additional 20 to 25 minutes or until fish flakes easily with fork.

Makes 4 servings with 252 calories and 2.2 grams fat each.

376. *Easy Popcorn Caramel Brittle*

¾ cup salted dry-roasted peanuts
1 cup miniature marshmallows

8 cups hot-air popped popcorn
1 cup water
3 cups sugar
½ teaspoon vanilla extract

1. In a large bowl combine peanuts, marshmallows, and popped corn, then set aside.

2. Combine water and sugar in a heavy, large dutch oven. Cook uncovered over medium-low heat, without stirring, until sugar dissolves (about 10 minutes). Without stirring, cover, increase heat to medium, and cook for 1 minute. Uncover and cook until amber, still without stirring (about 12 more minutes).

3. Remove from heat, stir in vanilla, and add popped-corn mixture. Working as quickly as possible, stir well and spread mixture into a 15″ × 10″ × 1″ jelly-roll pan coated with cooking spray. After it cools completely break it into pieces. Store in an airtight container.

Makes 12 1-ounce servings with 120 calories and 2.1 grams fat each.

377. *Energizing Fruit Slush*

5 cups water
1¾ cups sugar
1 6-ounce can frozen lemonade, thawed
1 6-ounce can frozen orange juice concentrate, thawed
3 medium bananas cut into 2-inch chunks
3 cups unsweetened pineapple juice
1 67.6-ounce bottle ginger ale

1. In a medium saucepan, bring water and sugar to a boil, reduce heat, simmer 4 to 5 minutes until sugar dissolves, then let cool. Process lemonade and orange juice concentrates with banana chunks in electric blender until smooth.

2. In a large freezable container combine sugar mixture with banana mixture and pineapple juice, cover, and freeze 8 hours.

3. To serve, let stand at room temperature for 45 minutes, place in a punch bowl, add chilled ginger ale, and stir until slushy.

Makes 14 1-cup servings with 167 calories and 0.1 gram fat each.

378. *Exciting Mashed Potatoes*

9 ounces potatoes, pared and cubed
¼ cup diced onion
1½ cloves garlic, chopped
⅛ cup skim milk
2 teaspoons margarine
Dash white pepper

1. Cook potatoes, onion, and garlic until potatoes are fork-tender (10 to 15 minutes) in 1½ quarts boiling water. While potatoes cook, combine milk, margarine, and pepper in a small nonstick saucepan and cook over low heat until margarine is melted. Keep warm and liquid over low heat.

2. Drain potato/onion mixture in a colander and transfer to a large mixing bowl. Mash using a mixer on low speed. Gradually increase mixer speed to high, add milk mixture, and continue beating until fluffy and light.

Makes 2 servings with 170 calories and 4 grams fat each.

379. *Fabulous Italian Figs*

2 tablespoons pine nuts, toasted
¼ cup minced candied mixed fruit
⅛ teaspoon ground cloves
18 whole dried Calimyrna figs
2 ounces semisweet chocolate, melted
1 ounce white chocolate, melted

1. In a small bowl combine pine nuts, mixed fruit, and cloves.

2. Preheat oven to 350 degrees. Trim stems from figs and cut each lengthwise, cutting to, but not through, the base of the fig. Carefully open each fig, press in 1 teaspoon of fruit mixture, and then press closed.

3. Bake 15 minutes, transfer to plate, drizzle chocolates over top, and chill 15 minutes to harden chocolate. Store in refrigerator.

Makes 6 servings (3 figs per serving) with 211 calories and 7.3 grams fat each.

380. *Fast and Flavorful Chicken Salad*

1 tablespoon chopped almonds
1½ pounds chicken breast, boned and skinned
½ cup sliced green onion
1 cup diagonally sliced celery
1 9-ounce jar commercial mango chutney
6 cups sliced and loosely packed romaine

1. To toast almonds, place on a baking sheet and bake at 350 degrees for 8 minutes or until toasted (watch them so they don't burn). Place a large nonstick skillet coated with nonstick spray over medium heat until hot. When skillet is hot cook chicken on each side 7 minutes, or until done, then remove. With a sharp knife slice chicken across grain into thin slices.

2. Line six individual plates with romaine. Combine chicken, onion, celery, almonds, and chutney in a large bowl and toss to coat. Spoon onto lettuce-lined plates and serve.

Makes 6 servings with 259 calories and 4.7 grams fat each.

381. *Favorite Buttermilk Dressing*

2 cups skim buttermilk, strained
½ cup red wine vinegar

1 teaspoon chervil
1 cup no-added-salt tomato juice
2 garlic cloves, minced
1 teaspoon basil

In a medium bowl whisk all ingredients together, transfer to screw-top container, and refrigerate.

Makes 40 1-tablespoon servings with 4 calories and 0 grams fat each.

382. *Favorite Butterscotch Cookies*

⅓ cup softened margarine
⅓ cup sugar
½ cup dark brown sugar, packed
2 egg whites
1 teaspoon vanilla extract
½ teaspoon baking soda
1¾ cups all-purpose flour
½ teaspoon salt
⅓ cup butterscotch morsels

1. In a large mixing bowl, use electric mixer to cream margarine. Gradually add sugars with mixer at medium speed until well blended. Beat in egg whites and vanilla. In a separate bowl combine baking soda, flour, and salt, then gradually add to creamed mixture, beating well after each addition. Stir in butterscotch morsels.

2. Preheat oven to 350 degrees. Coat a baking sheet with nonstick spray, mold mixture into roughly 32 balls, and place on baking sheets. Bake for 11 minutes, then remove from sheet and cool on rack.

Makes 32 servings with 74 calories and 2.4 grams fat each.

383. *Greatest Grapefruit Caesar Salad in the Land*

2 tablespoons skim milk
¼ cup grapefruit juice

½ cup low-fat cottage cheese
¼ teaspoon black pepper
2 anchovies
2 tablespoons extra-virgin olive oil
2 cloves garlic
1 ounce grated Parmesan cheese
1 head romaine
6 ounces cooked and chilled shrimp
12 ounces grapefruit segments, peeled

In a blender container place first seven ingredients and process at high speed. Fold in Parmesan and chill for 1 hour. Tear lettuce and toss with shrimp and grapefruit in a large salad bowl. Toss salad with chilled dressing and serve.

Makes 6 servings with 115 calories and 2.9 grams fat each.

384. *Honey Salad*

2 cups chopped apples
1 tablespoon lemon juice
½ cup sliced green grapes
½ cup finely diced celery
⅓ cup chopped walnuts
2 tablespoons honey
¼ cup fat-free mayonnaise

Coat apples with lemon juice to retard browning. Stir together all ingredients and serve.

Makes 8 servings with 79 calories and 2.6 grams fat each.

385. *Honeydew-Heaven Slush*

¼ cup confectioners sugar
½ honeydew melon, cubed (5 cups)
¼ cup bottled lime juice
2 cups crushed ice
Honeydew slices for garnish
Mint sprigs

In an electric blender container combine sugar, melon, and lime juice and process until smooth. Gradually add ice until smooth and serve immediately with honeydew slices and mint sprigs as garnish.

Makes 4 half-cup servings with 36 calories and 0 grams fat each.

386. *Jamaican Pineapple Treat*

2 cups chopped fresh pineapple
¾ cup chilled nonfat evaporated milk
¼ cup whipping cream
¼ tablespoon powdered sugar
1 teaspoon vanilla
4 tablespoons flaked coconut

1. Place pineapple in strainer for 12 minutes. Meanwhile, whip milk and cream in a large bowl with an electric mixer to soft peak. Gradually add sugar to taste. Add vanilla and continue beating to hard peak.

2. Chill pineapple and whipped milk mixture separately. To serve, fold pineapple into milk mixture, spoon into chilled dessert bowls, and garnish with coconut.

Makes 4 servings with 173 calories and 5.8 grams fat each.

387. *Leek/Cucumber Salad*

¼ teaspoon dried tarragon
⅛ teaspoon salt
⅛ teaspoon white pepper
3 tablespoons nonfat Italian dressing
1 cup sliced leeks
2 medium cucumbers, sliced thin
½ cup halved cherry tomatoes

In a shaker container, combine tarragon, salt, pepper, and Italian dressing, then set aside. Toss together leeks, cucumbers, and tomatoes in a 2-quart salad bowl, then pour liquid mixture over top just prior to serving.

Makes 4 servings with 40 calories and 3 grams fat each.

388. *Light and Tasty Lorraine*

1 package refrigerated breadstick dough (7 ounces)
1½ cups onion slivers
6 slices turkey bacon, chopped
¾ cup low-fat/low-salt Swiss cheese (3 ounces)
1 cup evaporated skim milk
2 eggs
2 egg whites
⅛ teaspoon ground nutmeg
Ground red pepper
2 teaspoons cornstarch

1. Preheat oven to 375 degrees. On a flat surface separate breadstick dough into strips, then coil and join strips together around and around in a concentric circle until you end up with an 8-inch flat circle. Using a rolling pin, roll this into a 13-inch circle and then place in a 9-inch quiche dish, fold edges under, and flute.

2. Coat a medium nonstick skillet with nonstick cooking spray and place over medium-high heat until hot. Add onion and bacon, then cook 10 minutes stirring frequently. Spread in prepared crust and top with cheese.

3. In an electric blender container combine milk with eggs and egg whites, nutmeg, pepper, and cornstarch. Blend until smooth. Pour blended mixture over cheese and bake for 35 minutes, or until a knife inserted in center comes out clean. Let stand 10 minutes and serve.

Makes 6 servings with 236 calories and 8.2 grams fat each.

389. *Light Herb Dip*

⅛ teaspoon celery seed
⅛ teaspoon caraway seed
⅛ cup chopped fresh dill
8 ounces nonfat yogurt
½ tablespoon grated onion
Fresh dill for garnish
1 steamed artichoke

1. Combine first five ingredients in a small bowl. Cover and chill several hours or overnight.

2. Top with a sprinkling of dill and serve as a dip for artichoke leaves.

Makes about 4 quarter-cup servings with 32 calories and 0 grams fat each.

390. *Light Pound Cake*

3 cups sugar
¾ cup margarine, softened
1⅓ cups egg substitute, thawed
1 teaspoon baking soda
1½ cups low-fat sour cream
¼ teaspoon salt
½ cup sifted cake flour
2 teaspoons vanilla extract

1. Preheat oven to 325 degrees. In a large mixing bowl, combine sugar with softened margarine and blend with an electric mixer at medium speed. Gradually add egg substitute while beating well.

2. In a small bowl combine baking soda with sour cream and set to the side. In another bowl combine salt and cake flour.

3. With mixer on low speed, add a little sour cream mixture to sugar/margarine cream bowl, then a little flour/salt mixture, then a little sour cream mixture until it's all combined. Stir in vanilla extract. For variety, you can substitute ingredients in Tips 391 to 395 for the vanilla.

4. Lightly coat a 10-inch tube pan with nonstick cooking spray and spoon the batter into it. Bake for 1 hour and 35 minutes, or until a wooden toothpick inserted into center comes out clean. Cool for 10 minutes, then remove cake from pan and let it cool further on a rack.

Makes 24 servings (1-inch slices) with 250 calories and 6.8 grams fat each.

391. *Almond Pound Cake.* Decrease vanilla extract to 1 teaspoon and add 1 teaspoon almond extract.

392. *Butter Rum Pound Cake.* Decrease vanilla extract to 1 teaspoon, and add 1 teaspoon butter flavoring and 1 teaspoon rum flavoring.

393. *Butter-Flavored Pound Cake.* Decrease vanilla extract to 1 teaspoon and add 1 teaspoon butter flavoring.

394. *Coconut Pound Cake.* Decrease vanilla extract to 1 teaspoon and add 1 teaspoon coconut flavoring.

395. *Lemon Pound Cake.* When you add the 2 teaspoons of vanilla extract, also add 1 teaspoon grated lemon zest (the outer yellow part of the rind).

396. *Manhattan Grilled Sandwich*

1 tablespoon reduced-calorie mayonnaise
1 teaspoon Dijon mustard
4 slices rye bread
2 slices Swiss-flavored nonfat processed cheese product
4 ounces low-salt smoked ham, sliced thin
1 cup thinly sliced green cabbage

1. In a small bowl stir together mayonnaise and mustard, spread over two bread slices, and top each slice with one slice cheese, 1 ounce ham, ½ cup cabbage, another 1 ounce ham, and top bread slice.

2. Spray a nonstick skillet with nonstick cooking spray and place over medium heat until hot. Cook sandwiches 3 minutes each side, or until golden.

Makes 2 servings with 276 calories and 6 grams fat each.

397. *No-Mayo Potato Salad*

3 pounds potatoes
3 hard-boiled egg whites
½ cucumber, peeled, seeded, and diced
½ cup diced green bell pepper
½ cup chopped green onion
¼ cup minced fresh parsley
1 cup diced celery
Dash white pepper
Dash Hungarian paprika
Dash garlic powder
1 tablespoon unsweetened apple juice concentrate, still frozen
1 to 2 tablespoons tarragon vinegar
⅔ cup nonfat yogurt
2 teaspoons Dijon mustard
½ teaspoon crushed celery seed

1. Steam, cool, skin, and then dice potatoes. Coarsely grate egg whites. Mix together diced potatoes, egg whites, cucumber, green pepper, onion, parsley, and celery. While stirring, mix in white pepper, paprika, and garlic powder.

2. In another bowl combine juice, vinegar, yogurt, mustard, and celery seed. Pour this over potato mixture and toss. Chill for 2 to 3 hours before serving.

Makes 10 servings with 114 calories and 3 grams fat each.

398. *Orange-Basil Salmon Steaks*

½ cup frozen orange juice concentrate, thawed
¼ cup dry white wine
¼ cup chopped parsley
2 tablespoons corn oil
2 teaspoons dried basil
1 teaspoon salt
¾ teaspoon freshly ground pepper
4 salmon steaks (about 1½ pounds)
Fresh kumquats (optional)

1. In a shallow baking dish combine orange juice concentrate, wine, parsley, oil, basil, salt, and pepper.

2. Add salmon steaks and coat well with marinade. Cover and let stand at room temperature for 1 hour, turning once at 30 minutes.

3. Prepare grill for cooking or preheat broiler. Remove steaks from marinade. Grill or broil 4 to 5 inches from heat 8 to 10 minutes or until desired doneness, carefully turning once and brushing with marinade. Garnish with kumquats, if desired.

Makes 4 servings with 320 calories and 14 grams fat each
(without kumquats).

399. *Outstanding Chicken Club*

2 tablespoons balsamic vinegar
2 tablespoons no-added-salt tomato juice
2 4-ounce chicken breast halves, skinned and boned
Dash freshly ground black pepper
4 slices turkey bacon
6 slices toasted light sourdough bread
1 tablespoon reduced-calorie mayonnaise
8 ¼-inch tomato slices
2 cups loosely packed torn romaine

1. In a shallow glass bowl, combine vinegar and tomato juice, then set aside.

2. Flatten each chicken piece by placing between two sheets of heavy-duty plastic wrap and using a rolling pin or meat mallet. Add the flattened chicken to the vinegar mixture. Marinate in refrigerator, covered, for at least 1 hour, turning chicken about every 20 minutes.

3. Spray a light coat of nonstick cooking spray onto a nonstick skillet and place over medium heat until hot. Remove chicken from marinade and discard marinade. When skillet is hot, add chicken and cook 2 minutes on each side or until done. Remove from skillet, sprinkle with pepper, set aside, and keep warm in a small covered ceramic or glass container.

4. Cook turkey bacon in microwave according to package directions. Cut each slice in half crosswise, set aside, and keep warm.

5. Spread two slices of bread with ¾ teaspoon mayonnaise each. Top each with one chicken breast half, two tomato slices, and ½ cup lettuce; cover with another slice of bread, and top each with four half-slices of bacon, two tomato slices, and ½ cup lettuce. On remaining slices of bread spread ¾ teaspoon mayonnaise, then place a slice on top of each sandwich. Cut in half and secure with toothpicks.

Makes 2 servings with 370 calories and 10.5 grams fat each.

400. *Oven Onion Rings*

2 medium yellow onions
2 teaspoons canola oil
5 tablespoons crushed corn flakes

1. Preheat oven to 450 degrees. Cut onions into thin slices and then separate into rings.

2. Combine onions with oil in a large bowl and stir to coat. Add crushed corn flakes and toss to coat.

3. Coat a nonstick baking sheet with nonstick cooking spray and spread onion mixture onto sheet. Bake until onion rings are brown and crispy, turning frequently (about 20 minutes).

Makes 2 servings with 136 calories and 5 grams fat each.

401. *Perfect Fruit Punch*

12 ounces frozen tangerine juice concentrate, thawed
2½ cups cold water
4 cups chilled cranberry juice cocktail
½ cup fresh lime juice
½ cup fresh lemon juice
1 cup peeled, diced mango
Lemon slices
Lime slices

In a large punch bowl combine tangerine juice with water, cranberry juice cocktail, lemon juice, and lime juice. Mix well and then stir in mango. Top with floating lemon and lime slices.

Makes 12 ¾-cup servings with 110 calories and 0.2 gram fat each.

402. *Pizzazz Corn Bread*

2½ tablespoons vegetable oil
¾ cup all-purpose flour
½ teaspoon baking soda
¾ teaspoon baking powder
¾ cup yellow cornmeal
1 teaspoon chili powder
½ teaspoon salt
1 cup plain nonfat yogurt
1 8¾-ounce can no-added-salt whole-kernel corn, drained

1 4-ounce can chopped green chile peppers, drained
1 lightly beaten egg
1 lightly beaten egg white

1. Preheat oven to 400 degrees. Coat a 9-inch cast-iron skillet with oil. Place in oven for 5 minutes to "season" and set aside. In a large bowl stir together flour, baking soda, baking powder, cornmeal, chili powder, and salt. In a separate bowl, combine yogurt, corn, peppers, and eggs. Make a well in the middle of dry ingredients, and pour yogurt mixture into well, then mix with dry ingredients until moistened.

2. Add hot oil from skillet to batter and stir to combine. Pour batter into skillet and bake at 400 degrees for 25 minutes. Serve warm.

Makes 12 servings with 118 calories and 3.7 grams fat each.

403. *Quick and Tasty Cauliflower Meal*

4 cups cauliflower florets, blanched
½ cup tomato sauce
1½ ounces part-skim mozzarella cheese, shredded
2 tablespoons grated Parmesan cheese

1. Preheat oven to 375 degrees. Coat a 9-inch glass pie plate with nonstick cooking spray. Place cauliflower in pie plate and spoon tomato sauce over top.

2. Combine cheeses in a small mixing bowl and sprinkle over top. Bake 15 minutes, or until cauliflower is thoroughly heated.

Makes 4 servings with 74 calories and 3 grams fat each.

404. *Salad Scrumptious Pizza*

8 ounces pizza dough
2 cups thinly sliced arugula
2 medium red onions, sliced thin and separated into rings
2 chopped plum tomatoes

2 cups thinly sliced radicchio
1 tablespoon balsamic vinegar
¼ teaspoon black pepper
¼ teaspoon salt
1 tablespoon plus 1 teaspoon extra-virgin olive oil
3 ounces fontina cheese, shredded

1. Heat oven to 475 degrees. Press dough into a 12-inch pizza pan coated with nonstick cooking spray. Prick dough surface with fork and bake 10 to 15 minutes or until golden. While dough is baking, toss together arugula, onion, tomatoes, and radicchio in a large bowl. Add vinegar, pepper, and salt, mix well, and let stand 15 minutes.

2. Spread radicchio mixture onto prebaked dough using slotted spoon. Drizzle oil evenly over top and sprinkle with cheese.

Makes 8 servings with 144 calories and 7 grams fat each.

405. *Sensational Sesame Chicken*

4 chicken breast halves, skinned
2 tablespoons low-sodium soy sauce
2 tablespoons all-purpose flour
3 tablespoons sesame seeds
¼ teaspoon salt
¼ teaspoon pepper
1 tablespoon melted low-calorie margarine

1. Preheat oven to 400 degrees. Coat chicken with soy sauce by rolling in a shallow dish and set aside. Combine flour, sesame seeds, and salt and pepper in a large zip-top plastic bag. Add chicken and shake to coat.

2. Coat a 13″ × 9″ × 2″ baking dish with cooking spray and place chicken inside. Drizzle chicken with margarine and bake at 400 degrees for 45 minutes.

Makes 4 servings with 223 calories and 8.2 grams fat each.

406. *Sesame-Healthy Granola*

1½ ounces whole-grain cereal squares
1 ounce pecans, chopped fine
3 ounces quick oats
1½ ounces rice, wheat, or oat bran
1 tablespoon sesame seeds
¼ cup honey
¼ cup frozen apple juice concentrate, thawed
1 tablespoon plus 1 teaspoon vegetable oil
½ teaspoon almond extract
4½ ounces mixed dried fruit, chopped
¼ teaspoon cinnamon
Nonfat strawberry yogurt (optional)

1. Preheat oven to 350 degrees. Stir together cereal squares, pecans, oats, bran, and sesame seeds in a medium-sized bowl. In a one-cup measure combine honey, juice concentrate, oil, and extract, then drizzle over oat mixture while stirring until crumbly.

2. Line a large baking sheet with foil. Spread mixture onto foiled pan and bake until lightly browned, 10 to 12 minutes, stirring every 5 minutes. Cool and stir in fruit and cinnamon. Serve with yogurt, if desired.

Makes 8 servings with 211 calories and 7 grams fat each
(without yogurt).

407. *Shrimp with Tomato Vinaigrette*

2 large lemons, sliced
4 quarts water
60 fresh medium uncooked shrimp, unpeeled
2 cups no-added-salt tomato juice
1½ tablespoons extra-virgin olive oil
½ cup clam juice
¼ cup white wine vinegar
1 tablespoon plus 1 teaspoon anchovy paste

2 cloves garlic, crushed
Dash white pepper
1 cup chopped yellow bell pepper
1 cup chopped green bell pepper
1 cup chopped tomato, unpeeled

1. In a large saucepan combine lemon slices with water and bring to a boil. Add shrimp and cook 3 to 5 minutes. Drain, rinse with cold tap water, and then devein and peel shrimp. Cover and chill shrimp.

2. In a medium-sized bowl combine tomato juice, olive oil, clam juice, vinegar, anchovy paste, garlic, and white pepper, then stir until blended. In a separate bowl, combine yellow and green pepper and tomato. Add pepper mixture to the tomato juice mixture. Cover and chill.

3. When ready to serve, put five shrimp into each of 12 shallow bowls and top each portion with ½ cup of the tomato juice and bell pepper mixture.

Makes 12 servings with 99 calories and 3.1 grams fat each.

408. *Snappy Mexican Snapper*

1 clove garlic, chopped fine
½ teaspoon salt
⅛ teaspoon ground red pepper
1 teaspoon cumin
¼ cup bottled lime juice
3 tablespoons finely chopped cilantro
2 tomatoes, chopped
⅓ cup seeded and finely chopped jalapeño
⅓ cup chopped onion
1½ pounds red snapper fillets

1. Stir together garlic, salt, red pepper, cumin, and lime juice in a small bowl. In a separate medium bowl stir together 2 tablespoons of this lime mixture (set the rest aside),

cilantro, tomatoes, jalapeño, and onion. Refrigerate salsa until you're ready to serve.

2. Preheat broiler. Arrange fish on broiler pan and brush top with remaining lime mixture. Broil 4 to 6 inches from heat for 4 minutes. Carefully turn fish and brush other side with lime mixture and repeat broiling 4 minutes, or until fish flakes easily with fork. Serve fish topped with salsa.

Makes 6 servings with 145 calories and 2 grams fat each.

409. *State of the Art Chicken Chili*

3 cloves garlic, minced
3 jalapeños, chopped
1 cup chopped green bell pepper
1½ cups chopped yellow onion
2 teaspoons cumin
½ teaspon dried oregano
2 tablespoons chili powder
1 cup water
2 cups chicken thigh meat, cut into bite-sized pieces
2 cups chicken breast meat, cut into bite-sized pieces
¼ teaspoon black pepper
½ teaspoon ground red pepper
1 tablespoon Dijon mustard
1 tablespoon Worcestershire sauce
1 14½-ounce can no-added-salt stewed tomatoes
1 13¾-ounce can no-added-salt chicken broth
1 12-ounce bottle reduced-calorie chili sauce
1 16-ounce can Great Northern beans
1¼ cups chopped purple onion
1¼ cups diced avocado
½ cup plus 2 tablespoons plain nonfat yogurt

1. Coat a dutch oven with nonfat cooking spray and place on medium heat until hot, then add garlic, jalapeño, green

pepper, and yellow onion. Sauté 5 to 6 minutes, add cumin, oregano, and chili powder, and cook 2 minutes. Add the water, chicken, black pepper, red pepper, Dijon, Worcestershire, tomatoes, chicken broth, and chili sauce. Bring to a boil, reduce heat, cover, and simmer 25 minutes.

2. Add beans and simmer 5 minutes. To serve, top each bowl with purple onion, avocado, and yogurt.

Makes 9 one-cup servings with 300 calories and 9.8 grams fat each.

410. *Superb Microwave Sauce "Hollandaise"*

¼ cup frozen egg substitute, thawed
1 tablespoon plus 1 teaspoon low-calorie margarine
½ teaspoon Dijon mustard
1 teaspoon lemon juice
Dash ground red pepper

1. In a one-cup microwave container combine egg substitute with margarine. Microwave on low for 1 minute until margarine softens, stirring once at 30 seconds.

2. Stir in mustard and juice and microwave on low for 3 minutes until thickened, stirring every 30 seconds. Stir in red pepper. If sauce curdles, just remove from microwave and blend in blender on low until smooth.

Makes 2 servings with 52 calories and 4 grams fat each.

411. *Superb Sweet Chicken*

2 chicken cutlets (¼ pound each)
2 teaspoons all-purpose flour
1 tablespoon soft low-calorie margarine
1 cup sliced mushrooms
1 small clove garlic, minced
1 cup chopped leeks
4 large plum tomatoes

2 tablespoons balsamic vinegar
2 tablespoons dry white table wine
1 tablespoon honey
1 tablespoon chopped fresh flat-leaf parsley

1. Dredge chicken cutlets in flour on a sheet of wax paper.

2. Melt margarine in a 9-inch nonstick skillet and add chicken. Cook over high heat until golden on each side (3 to 4 minutes). Set aside.

3. Combine mushrooms, garlic, and leeks in the same skillet, then sauté over medium heat about 2 minutes until leeks are crisp-tender. Blanch, peel, seed, and chop tomatoes, then mix with vinegar, wine, honey, and parsley and bring to a boil.

4. After mixture reaches a boil, reduce heat and add chicken to the skillet. Let chicken simmer in skillet covered for about 3 minutes or until thoroughly heated.

Makes 2 servings with 273 calories and 6 grams fat each.

412. *Super-Easy Chinese Chicken*

3 chicken thighs, skinned
3 chicken drumsticks, skinned
3 chicken breast halves, skinned
½ cup packed brown sugar
½ cup reduced-calorie ketchup
2 tablespoons white vinegar
½ teaspoon garlic powder
1 tablespoon instant onion flakes
½ teaspoon low-sodium seasoned salt
¼ cup low-sodium soy sauce

1. Place chicken pieces in a 13″ × 9″ × 2″ baking dish. Combine remaining ingredients, stir, and pour over chicken.

2. Bake at 350 degrees uncovered for 1½ hours. Baste every 25 minutes, and turn chicken over after 45 minutes.

Makes 9 servings with 208 calories and 3.6 grams fat each.

413. *Ultra-Fast Breakfast*

2 tablespoons frozen orange juice concentrate
¾ cup plain low-fat yogurt
1 tablespoon wheat germ
1 piece fresh fruit cut into chunks or ½ cup fresh berries

In a blender container mix juice concentrate, yogurt, and wheat germ. Stir in fruit. Process until smooth.

Makes 1 serving with 327 calories and 1.8 grams fat.

414. *Vanilla-Cherry Soda*

½ cup cold water
1 packet low-calorie vanilla-flavored dairy drink mix
6 ice cubes
1 cup low-calorie black cherry soda
½ cup vanilla ice milk
2 maraschino cherries

1. In an electric blender container process the water and drink mix on low speed until combined. With blender on high add ice cubes one at a time until mixture is desired thickness. Add soda and process on low speed.

2. Pour half into each of two 12-ounce glasses and add ¼ cup ice milk to each. Top with cherry.

Makes 2 servings with 84 calories and 1 gram fat each.

415. *World's Best Light Cucumber Dip*

½ cup minced cucumber
½ cup finely chopped smoked turkey breast
1¼ cups nonfat yogurt
¼ teaspoon dill weed

Combine all ingredients in a small bowl, cover, and chill.

Makes 1 serving with 237 calories and 2.6 grams fat.

416. *Yogurt-Pudding Chocolate Sponge Cake*

1 teaspoon double-acting baking powder
¾ cup cake flour
4 large eggs, at room temperature
⅓ cup sugar
1 envelope instant reduced-calorie chocolate pudding and pie-filling mix
1 cup plain low-fat yogurt

1. Preheat oven to 400 degrees. Coat a 15″ × 10″ × 1″ jelly-roll pan with nonstick cooking spray, then line it with a sheet of parchment or wax paper. Coat paper again with nonstick spray and set aside.

2. Sift together baking powder and flour on a sheet of wax paper and set aside.

3. In a large bowl beat eggs with electric mixer on high speed, then gradually add sugar, 1 tablespoon at a time, until volume doubles. Fold in the flour mixture.

4. Carefully spread batter mixture in paper-lined jelly-roll pan, and bake in center of oven 5 to 8 minutes or until golden. The top should bounce back when touched lightly with your finger.

5. For icing, in blender combine pudding mix and yogurt and blend until smooth. Invert cake onto work surface and remove paper from cake.

6. Cut crosswise into quarter-slices, then spread a quarter of the icing over each quarter-section of the cake. Stack the four layers on a serving plate with the icing side up.

Makes 8 servings with 150 calories and 3 grams fat each.

417. *Your Best Russian Dressing*

> 2 hard-boiled egg whites, chopped
> 1 cup nonfat yogurt
> ¼ cup no-added-salt tomato sauce
> ½ teaspoon onion powder
> ¼ cup diced green bell pepper
> Dash Tabasco
> Dash garlic powder
> Dash Hungarian paprika
> Dash thyme
> Fresh parsley for garnish

> In a medium bowl, whisk all ingredients together, then store in refrigerator in screw-top container. Serve with fresh parsley as garnish.

Makes 24 1-tablespoon servings with 7 calories and 0.2 gram fat each.

9.

Fitness Tips[8]

Getting Started

418. Energize your routine with these activity boosters. Try Tips 419 through 429 next time you feel lazy. You may be pleasantly surprised at the results:

419. *Use what coaches call "the five-minute rule."* For instance, say you are lying on the couch watching TV, have just finished dinner, and are tired. You look over and see your walking shoes by the door, but you just don't feel like lacing them up and walking tonight. What you can do is tell yourself this, "Okay, I'll try it for just five minutes, and if it doesn't work, I'll quit."

420. *Exercise for better sex.* Remind yourself that people who exercise regularly not only have sex more often, but also enjoy their sex more!

421. *Use a friendly rivalry.* Find a friendly adversary to match for total exercise time each week or month. Call each other at least weekly to keep each other motivated, and to motivate the person who has less total exercise time.

---

[8]It's always a good idea to consult your physician before you begin any new exercise program.

422. *Put your money where your mouth is.* In a Michigan State University study, 97 percent of people who bet $40 they could stick with their exercise program for six months did so, while only 20 percent of those who didn't bet succeeded. Betting money on yourself is definitely worth a try.

423. *Understand how critical exercise is to permanent weight control.* If you were to track a group of people for a year after they lost weight, *90 percent* of those who kept their weight off would be exercising regularly, according to a study of a large HMO published in the *American Journal of Clinical Nutrition* in 1990. This is very compelling proof of the power of exercise. Next time you don't feel like exercising, remind yourself that you're committed to lifestyle change and are doing something positive toward that goal.

424. *Sleep in your exercise clothing.* If you exercise in the morning, then go to sleep with your sweat clothing on and have your shoes and socks ready by the door to make it as easy as possible for you to exercise.

425. *Put together a selection of exercise music you find motivating.*

426. *Focus on how you feel when you're done.* Avoid saying to yourself such things as, "Oh, I feel rotten and it's raining and cold, and I really don't want to go for a walk." Instead, focus on how you're going to feel when you're done by saying something like, "I always feel so confident, relaxed, and happy after I've finished exercising, and followed it with a nice hot shower. I can't wait to sit down with a good book and some raspberry tea afterward, feeling clean, healthy, and relaxed."

427. *Exercise because you enjoy being alive.* People with low levels of physical activity may be more than twice as likely to die earlier than people with moderate physical activity levels.

428. *Exercise for a stronger and healthier heart.* It's an absolute myth that humans are born with X number of heartbeats and when

they're used up you die. Your heart is a muscle that grows stronger and more efficient with exercise.

429. *Exercise to improve your performance and attitude at work.* Exercise can make you more productive and energetic at work, and also give you a sense that your work is less boring than when you don't exercise.

430. **Choose the best time for you to exercise.** To improve the quantity and quality of your exercise, exercise at the time of day that's best for you. Once you've established when you're going to exercise, exercise at roughly the same time every day. Your body responds to habit. Be flexible, though, and don't hesitate to exercise at another time if you can't fit your regular time into your schedule. You can use the guidelines in Tips 431 to 435 to discover your optimal time of day for exercise:

431. *The morning is a good time to exercise if you're constantly finding it difficult to make time for exercise.* When you exercise first thing in the morning, it's much less likely that a big problem will surface that will prevent you from exercising.

432. *The afternoon is a good time to exercise for people who want to perform at their absolute best.* By this time of day your joints are flexible and your metabolism is up and running, so you're ready to exercise at peak performance.

433. *The late afternoon is a good time to exercise if you want to control your appetite for dinner.* It's proven that exercise curbs the appetite. (If you exercise and feel increased hunger, it's your mind talking rather than your body.)

434. *If stress is a big problem for you, the early evening is a good time to exercise.* After all your problems pile up during the day, it's wonderful to get out and release the day's tension through exercise.

435. *Take it easy when you exercise late at night.* Late-evening exercise will accelerate your metabolism, which may make it difficult for you to sleep. Some people can exercise late at night, take a hot bath, and then sleep like a baby. Others can't. See what works best for you.

436. **Use your big muscles for a better workout.** Activities that use the big muscles of your lower body (thighs and buttocks) will give you a better calorie-burning workout than activities that don't.

437. **Realize that any exercise is better than no exercise.** You don't have to exercise a certain magical amount in order for your exercise to have value. Yes, as discussed in Part I it's best if you exercise in blocks of at least 15 minutes, but that doesn't mean if you exercise less you won't receive any benefits. You most definitely will! Anything, anything at all, that makes you more active counts.

438. **Set a goal of six months to overcome feelings of embarrassment or inadequacy.** When you first start your aerobic exercise program, you may feel embarrassed or inadequate at your lack of ability. Just keep in mind that you're not alone. Observation of thousands of people starting aerobic exercise programs by researchers at the Institute for Aerobics Research in Dallas, Texas, has revealed that nearly everyone starts out with one or the other of these feelings. Generally speaking, people starting an aerobic exercise program will experience the following stages:

    - agony
    - discouragement
    - determination
    - at roughly six weeks, first small successes
    - 50 percent quit between the third and sixth months
    - success at roughly six months
    - smugness

    Notice that the final stage is smugness! When, six months after they've succeeded, you ask people who started out feeling fat, wheezy, foolish, and awkward how they got started, you'll probably get a one-liner such as, "It was pretty tough, but I did it." Then they'll go into a long discourse about how wonderful exercise is! You see, what typically happens after six months is you forget all the difficulty you had at first and become immersed in all the good life-enhancing feelings exercise gives you. When you make your next attempt at an exercise program, promise yourself you'll stay with it, be completely honest with yourself, and try your very best for six full months. If you do this, the chances are very good you'll finally overcome any negative feelings you may have about exercise, and emerge a new person who truly enjoys and looks forward to exercise.

439. **Stress variety if you're over 40.** Post-exercise muscle repair takes longer in people over 40. If you want to work out at a moderate or high intensity every day, then the solution is to work different muscle groups on different days. For instance, you could swim one day and then jog the next. After a tough workout, give the muscle group you worked roughly 48 hours to rest before exercising that specific group again. Also, if you're over 40 and just starting to exercise, don't think you're too old. Many seniors achieve record levels of fitness after starting in their 60s, 70s, or even 80s. Our reflexes slow and we lose some flexibility with age, but our cardio-vascular fitness can be maintained at very high levels until old age. One man more than 100 years old even climbed Mt. Fuji! Check with your doctor first, start out easy, gradually work your way up to a moderate level of exercise, and stress a variety of exercises, and you'll do much to enhance your life and weight control at any age.

440. **Prevent boredom.** It's human nature for adults to become bored when doing the same thing over and over again. Experiment with Tips 441 through 445 to liven up your exercise:

441. *Teach someone else.* Through a student's eyes you can capture the excitement you felt when you first started your activity. This

excitement, combined with the challenge of trying to know your activity well enough to teach it, can be very motivating.

442. *Become an expert.* Read books and magazines, and attend lectures. Challenge yourself by becoming an expert on your activity.

443. *Enjoy a variety of activities and buy mostly used equipment to make them affordable.* It's time consuming at first to learn a variety of activities, but it will pay off over the long term. For instance, when you've become tired of mountain biking, or the weather's bad, you'll be able to swim instead. If you don't feel like swimming, you'll go dancing. You can easily buy used clothing and equipment because people are always starting new activities and then quitting them. Also, be sure to borrow or rent equipment when trying a new activity. Don't buy equipment until you're sure you'll enjoy it.

444. *Explore organized competition.* Friendly competition can be fun and a great way to motivate yourself. Participate in timed walks, cycling events, or swims. Contact the organization for the activity you're interested in by locating its address in Tips 594 through 671. Ask about local competitions in your area. You could also ask the salesperson who specializes in your activity at your local sports store or contact local health club and pool managers. If you participate in an activity that requires more than one person such as tennis, handball, or basketball, then try to compete with people of similar ability. If you're better than everyone else, you won't burn as many calories as your competitors.

445. *Try swimming for a very different workout experience.* To jump into a pool of water is to escape the world of gravity and noise you live in all day long, and to immerse yourself in a fluid medium that's cool, sensual, and exhilarating. For more on swimming, see Tip 537.

446. **Don't damage your hair with rubber bands.** Try a clip, headbands, or an old baseball cap for style and hair protection.

447. **Don't expect miracles from chromium picolinate.** Research at the U.S. Department of Agriculture Human Nutrition Research Center in Grand Forks, North Dakota, proved "chromium picolinate has *no effect* on building muscle, reducing body fat, changing body composition, decreasing weight or increasing strength." This so-called fitness product is an aggressively marketed scam.

448. **Realize that only athletes need wonder drinks.** Plain ol' water is by far the best thing to drink before, during, and after a workout. People selling wonder drinks would like us to believe that a huge amount of potassium and sodium is lost when we exercise. For a normal workout such as an aerobics class, however, this simply isn't true. If you reach the point where you're training at high intensity for 60 or more minutes several times a week, as a marathon runner would, then drinks such as Gatorade can be helpful. For most people, however, they are unnecessary.

449. **Don't think exercise as an adult is like exercise in high school.** You may have hated your gym teacher. You may have hated running, getting all sweaty, and going to class smelling like a pig. You may have hated everything about gym and dreaded it like the plague on days you had to go. If this describes you, you're in for a big surprise. Go try an aerobics class for starters. You should find exciting music and everyone pulling together and having fun.

450. **Make certain you choose a health club that's right for you.** *Consumer's Digest* reports that only one person in five who joins a health club will still be using the club at least twice a week a year later! This is unfortunate, since health clubs are an excellent means for people to achieve a healthy fitness level. Many people find the encouragement to exercise and social contact they receive at a health club very motivating. Tips 451 through 464 are designed to help you select a club that's right for you:

451. *Location, location, location.* You can narrow the number of clubs from which you choose right away by making a list of clubs that

are near work, home, or an area in which you run a lot of errands daily.

452. **Equipment, facilities, and services.** Find out which clubs on your list have the right equipment, facilities, and services. For instance, if you like to swim, then obviously you're going to want a club with a nice pool and showers. If you have children, you're going to want a club with quality child care. Don't forget to look at community centers and your local YMCA.

453. **What is the club's square-footage-to-membership ratio?** This is the total square footage divided by the number of members. The lower the number, the more crowded the center will be. You want your club's ratio to be 10:1 or higher. That's equal to 10 square feet per member.

454. **Does this club have a membership ceiling?** Will the club limit its membership if it reaches a certain number of members? If the club does have a membership ceiling, then divide the square footage by the membership ceiling and you can get an idea of how crowded the club will be when it's filled. Again, you want the ratio to be 10:1 or higher.

455. **What hours is the club open?** Make sure they're convenient for you.

456. **Are the equipment and facilities in good repair and easy to use?** Check everything you'll be using to see if it works. Also, make sure machines aren't crammed against walls or stuffed so close to each other they're difficult to use.

457. **What will it cost?** Include annual dues, initiation fees, and other expenses such as parking or child care. Is the equipment, social contact, and support the club provides worth the cost?

458. **Do you get special discounts?** Clubs may have discounts for seniors, students, or people who can work out during off-peak hours, which are usually 9:00 A.M. to 4:00 P.M.

459. *Is the club clean?* Make an unscheduled visit and check the whirlpool, locker rooms, and saunas to see if they're clean.

460. *Do the members like working out here?* Ask other members about the club's positives and negatives.

461. *What kind of clientele does the club have?* Ask this question, and during your visit look around to see what kind of people are in the club. Are these the kind of people with whom you want to exercise?

462. *Does the club belong to any associations?* Associations have standards that help to regulate clubs. Generally the best clubs will belong to the Association of Quality Clubs, abbreviated IRSA. Other associations include the Association of Physical Fitness Centers, most of which are Bally clubs, and a newer association called the National Health Club Association.

463. *What are the qualifications of the club's staff?* Do they have the appropriate education and certification?

464. *Choose a center and test it for a week through a trial membership.* Don't prepay any amount before you've tested a club! Use this time to talk further to members and to make sure the club operates the way you want it to during the times you'll be working out. If you don't like it after you've tested it, then try your second choice. If it turns out you don't like any health clubs, then that's fine. Health clubs aren't for everyone.

465. **Stretch to prevent injuries.** Try to make stretching a part of your workout mentality. Look forward to stretching. It's a wonderful time to psyche yourself for a workout or wind down after you've finished. Stretching varies from activity to activity. Read books or magazine articles, or ask a coach or trainer which stretches are best for your sport or activity. The classic book on the subject is Bob Anderson's *Stretching*, available at bookstores. In general, stretching should be done at a very relaxed pace. Stretch carefully

and without any bouncing motion. In addition, keep in mind the general points listed in Tips 466 to 472:

466. *Activity stretch.* A good warm-up and cool-down when you're first starting is to perform your activity slowly and easily for five minutes before and after the intense part of your workout. For instance, if you walk, swim, or cycle, then simply walk, swim, or cycle slowly and easily for five minutes before and after the intense part of your workout.

467. *Take it easy.* When a muscle is forced, it tends to fight back and resist. It may even pull or tear. To avoid "fight back," stretch your muscles slowly to the point of mild sensation and then hold. When you feel as if you could hold the stretch indefinitely without pain, you know you're not overstretching.

468. *Breathe deeply.* Take a deep breath and gradually let it out as you slowly reach to stretch.

469. *Take your time.* Do your stretches thoroughly and perform a consistent routine. Introduce new stretches gradually.

470. *Don't overstretch.* Too much stretching can do more harm than good.

471. *Don't aggravate.* Avoid stretches that aggravate preexisting conditions. You don't want to aggravate knee or back pain in particular.

472. *No injured or sore muscles.* Don't stretch muscles that are injured or sore. Take it easy on these muscles until they're completely healed.

473. **Remember the rule for an exercise lapse.** If you stop exercising for a time, as a general rule, the amount of time you didn't exercise should equal the amount of time you spend getting back to the level at which you last exercised. For instance, if you stopped walking for five weeks, then you'd want to take five weeks to get back to your previous level of activity. This is a general guideline.

If you're older or sedentary, you may want to take more time. If you're young, if you're physically fit, or if you've been participating in your activity regularly for more than a year, then you may want to take less time.

474. Wear comfortable exercise apparel. The bottom line on exercise apparel is that you should wear whatever makes you most comfortable. Aerobic exercise provides the same benefits whether you're wearing an old sweatshirt or the latest fabric. Try Tips 475 through 481:

475. *Layering.* It helps to layer your clothing in cold weather by wearing a T-shirt, several sweatshirts, and a Windbreaker. This way, after you've warmed up, you can take off a layer and tie it around your waist or stuff it into a backpack.

476. *Shoes.* Safe and comfortable footwear is crucial to a number of aerobic activities and is the one piece of exercise apparel on which you should be willing to spend a little extra money if necessary. Whether you walk, jog, or hike, take an old pair of shoes to a shoe department, find a knowledgeable and patient salesperson, and spend an afternoon selecting a good pair of shoes. It's important to take your old shoes because the wear pattern on them will help the salesperson select a new pair with characteristics that will be right for you.

477. *Running and cycling shorts.* Running shorts should have a generous side cut to maximize freedom of movement and should be lightweight, with a wicking comfort liner. Cycling shorts should be of lightweight yet durable fabric such as Lycra spandex/Supplex nylon or cotton/Lycra spandex, with a multi-panel, wicking crotch lining or panel for comfort, and aerodynamic cut for close, no-chafe fit.

478. *Cycling top.* At your discretion a cycling top can be either cut loose or form fitting, but should be lightweight and have moisture management properties.

479. *Woman's sport top or bra.* A woman's sport top or bra should have wide straps, few metal parts, and, for those women who need them, cups. Moisture management is also critical, since sweat can cause chafing around the nipple area.

480. *Foul weather suit.* Choose foul weather gear that is water- and wind-resistant, with calf zippers, ventilated back, and mesh or polypropylene fabric liner.

481. *Swimsuit.* Women should choose a biomechanical swimsuit cut to fit a swimmer's body, with a secure shoulder-strap system and a lightweight, quick-drying Lycra spandex and nylon (Antron, Supplex) fabric blend. Men should look for the same fabrics and opt for a close-fitting suit with a biomechanical cut and a drawstring. It's amazing how much a baggy suit impedes performance in the water.

482. **Create a workout that's right for you.** To personalize your workout, write out a list of features you want your ideal exercise to have, taking into consideration your current physical condition. Pick something you can do right away at your present pace. Also, decide whether you enjoy working out by yourself or with others, and choose activities you think you'll enjoy, that are accessible, and that provide the workout you want. For example, maybe you prefer to work out by yourself. You like low-impact activities. You want it to be aerobic to maximize fat burning, but at the same time use major muscle groups to tone your body. You want to be able to do it all year round, and you want it to be fun! Impossible? To find out, first go to the library and read about everything from square dancing to martial arts. Then, using the list of features you made earlier, find the activities that match most closely all your desired characteristics, the exercise that would be best for you. In this example, your activities could be cross-country skiing, using a cross-country ski machine, and in-line skating. All three offer a fun workout you can do yourself whenever you want, work the major muscle groups, and are aerobic. You can work out at home

on a cross-country ski machine when you're pressed for time. You can go in-line skating outdoors in the summer and ski in the winter. You've done it! You've personalized your workout.

Body Shaping

483. **Add exercise to changes in diet to produce a beautiful body shape.** To avoid transforming yourself from a big formless shape into a small formless shape, you should perform weight-bearing exercises. Adding these exercises to your aerobic workout will make your body as beautiful as possible and won't necessarily require much time or money. For instance, you could walk to receive an aerobic workout that's simultaneously a weight-bearing exercise for your lower body and, when it's convenient, work your arms using light dumbbells as discussed in Tips 486 to 489. You could do a dumbbell workout while your pasta boils, and then walk after dinner. You could do some push-ups when you first wake up, and then go for a 15-minute walk. You could keep a set of light dumbbells in a drawer at work, and then easily perform a 10-minute dumbbell workout during your lunch break, just before you leave, or just after you arrive. You could use a cross-country skiing or rowing machine each evening, or learn how to play tennis, squash, or handball, rock climb, kayak, row, cross-country ski, be a gymnast, or swim, and never lift a dumbbell at all, since these activities tone muscles in your upper body.

484. **Tighten your tush.** Don't spot exercise and expect miracles. Spot exercise will tone the muscles in the area you're working, but it won't get rid of the ugly flab. As you may know, women store their extra fat in certain locations on their bodies: hips, thighs, and behind the upper arms. Consequently the only way to get rid of fat on your tush is to reduce the amount of fat in your entire body. In other words, by reducing your *total body fat*, you'll reduce the fat on your tush. Aerobic activities such as swimming, running, walking, hiking, cycling, aerobic dancing, or cross-country skiing

maximize fat burning and so reduce the fat deposited in your hips, while also toning your buttocks and thighs. Don't waste another minute or dollar searching for a miracle exercise or exercise gadget that will tone your tush in minutes. The only miracles that will produce a tight tush are time and commitment. Be honest with yourself, put in the time and effort, and it will happen.

485. **Understand that thigh cream is not the answer to your prayers.** Revlon's Ultima II ProCollagen anti-cellulite body complex had the dubious distinction of winning the *Healthy Weight Journal*'s 1994 Slim Chance Award for worst product. Neither the American Medical Association nor the Food and Drug Administration recognizes cellulite as a medical problem. The much-advertised and discussed "medical research" used to support thigh-reducing cream was based only on 11 women and evidently didn't consider such important factors as hormonal swings, water displacement, muscle changes, and exercise! Cellulite is truly nothing more than a pseudoscientific quack term for fat. It's pockets of fat stored under the skin. The dreaded honeycomb pattern emerges because of two phenomena. Either your fat cells grow and push up against the skin, producing a bulge next to the fibrous cord that holds the skin, or, as your skin loses elasticity with age, it tightens around the fat pockets, resulting in the same kind of bulge. In women, these connective cords that hold the skin run parallel, rather than crisscross as they do in men. This makes women more susceptible to cellulite formations. Some treatments, such as paraffin masks, massages, or other salon techniques, may bring a very temporary change by squeezing fluid out of the cellulite area. This effect, however, doesn't last. The best strategy to reduce or prevent these fat deposits is to exercise aerobically to reduce your body's fat deposits, and to perform specific exercises that will tone the muscles in the area with which you're concerned.

486. **Tone your upper arms.** Exercise aerobically to reduce the fat deposited in your upper arms, and also perform the exercises listed in Tips 487 through 489 to make your arms strong and firm.

Keep in mind that building your shoulder muscles makes your waist appear smaller. If you haven't worked your upper arms in a while, it may take one or two months before you start to notice a much firmer upper arm:

487. *A supinated dumbbell curl works best for your biceps.* This is a complex label for a simple exercise. Here's how to do it. Grab your dumbbells (use light weight if you're a beginner) and stand erect with your feet shoulder-width apart and your knees slightly bent. Let your arms hang naturally, with the palms of your hands (holding dumbbell) facing your thighs. Keeping your back straight, with one arm move your dumbbell up in an arc and rotate slowly until the palm of your hand faces your shoulder. Now slowly lower your dumbbell in an arc and rotate until your palm ends up back where it started facing your thigh. Be sure to lower your arm completely before you start with your other arm. If you're good at it, you can do both arms at the same time. Just be sure to do it slowly, evenly, and as naturally as possible. Your ultimate goal is four sets of 15, 12, 10, and 6 to 8 repetitions at least three times per week.

488. *For your triceps, do overhead dumbbell presses and push-ups.* Grab a lightweight dumbbell and sit with good posture on a firm bench or low-back chair. Keep your torso erect and your feet flat on the floor. Raise the dumbbell up until your arm is fully extended straight over your head with your upper arm as close to your ear as possible. Your raised arm should be slightly bent at the elbow. Your other arm should be resting palm down on your opposite thigh. Now gradually lower the dumbbell in a natural arc down behind your head without moving your elbow. Keep your elbow stationary. Raise the dumbbell back up to your starting position and you've just done your first overhead dumbbell press. Repeat with the other arm. (Be sure to use a dumbbell and not a straight bar whenever possible. A straight bar will let you isolate muscle groups better, but there's also a good chance you'll over-work those groups or strain a joint or tendon. A straight bar

doesn't allow for natural enough movements.) Your ultimate goal is four sets of 15, 12, 10, and 6 to 8 repetitions at least three times per week. Again, focus on natural, slow, and fluid movements. Relaxing music might help.

Another good exercise for your triceps is the convenient and effective push-up. Do push-ups with your knees on the floor, your back straight, and hands slightly farther apart than your shoulders. Or, if you'd rather, you can also do them standing up, leaning at an angle against either a wall or counter top. Stand at arm's length facing a wall or counter top. Place both hands flat against the wall or counter top and slightly farther apart than shoulder-width. Keeping your feet flat, and your back straight, bend your arms and lower yourself toward the wall or counter top and then back up again. Try to work up to four sets of 30, 20, 15, and 12 repetitions at least three times a week.

489. *To make your routine easier:*

- Have a light set of dumbbells in visual sight near or in the kitchen at all times. In the 10 to 12 minutes it takes for most pasta to boil, you could finish working either your biceps or triceps.
- Have dumbbells by the telephone. You can work out while you talk on the phone.
- Have dumbbells in the television room, and work out while you watch television.
- Have dumbbells by your bed, and workout before you do anything else in the morning.

490. Flatten your tummy. Since belly fat poses a much greater danger to your health than hip or thigh fat, keeping your belly as lean as possible is very important. To do this, exercise aerobically to reduce the fat deposited on your tummy, and perform the following safe and effective abdominal workout to tone your tummy. The exercise is officially called ab curling. Lie flat on the floor and, keeping your knees bent and your arms across your chest, rise off the floor slowly, curling up each vertebra separately until you reach a 45-degree angle (look in a mirror or ask someone to watch when you're first starting). When you're at a 45-degree angle, your lower back should still be on the floor. Now lower yourself slowly back to the floor. That's it. After you become stronger, try keeping your stomach flexed even when you're on the floor. Also, try twisting to the right on the way up with one repetition, and then to the left on the way up with the next repetition. This will tone even more of your stomach area. The key is to keep your lower back firmly on the floor at all times. This way you don't involve weak back muscles that could be injured. You also want to keep your arms across your chest. Don't place your hands behind your neck. When you put your hands behind your neck there's a tendency to pull on your neck to lift yourself up. This could damage your neck muscles. You could try this exercise first thing in the morning, while watching television, or while listening to music.

491. **Use a bath towel to tone your tummy.** You don't have to spend a lot of money on weird gadgets that make doing sit-ups more comfortable. You don't even have to buy an expensive exercise mat. To do sit-ups at home, just grab an old, fairly thick towel and lay it on a carpeted floor. The carpeting has padding under it that, when combined with the towel, creates more than enough padding for your sit-ups. This strategy is terrific because it keeps you from slip-sliding around. The towel does this by absorbing sweat and creating friction between itself and the carpet. Slip-sliding is a troublesome problem associated with expensive rubberized or vinyl mats.

492. **Jump rope to work your whole body in minutes.** Jumping rope is a very intense exercise that will work your whole body in just 20 minutes. If you are starting and are sedentary, the first thing you should do is check with your health-care professional. Once you're ready, start by jumping in place for five minutes two times a day without a rope. If you can't do it for five minutes, then take breaks. After a week or so of just jumping around, you're ready

to try it with a rope. At first start slowly, then gradually increase the number of jumps you do each minute until you're performing about 70 to 100 jumps per minute. When you're done, warm your legs down with some walking. Drink plenty of fluid, eat right, and don't overdo it, otherwise you might get some calf-muscle cramping. It's definitely worth spending the time learning to jump rope. It's a refreshing change of pace from other workouts, it's cheap, it's easy to take with you on a trip, and it's fun. A change of scenery can make it even more enjoyable. Try the beach boardwalk, a park, the mountains, or different places around your home.

493. **Flex whenever possible.** While standing in line at the grocery store, sitting at work or at a red light, or watching television, gently but firmly tighten and then relax your abdomen or buttocks over and over again for a quick and convenient workout. These little motions will help to strengthen your musculature.

494. **Buy quality home exercise equipment you'll use.** Consumer demand for home gym equipment has skyrocketed over the past five years. The market has responded by providing literally hundreds of different exercise gizmos and gadgets, all purporting to burn the most fat with the least effort. How do you find the best home exercise machine for your dollar? After spending many months trying endless pieces of equipment and reading consumer guides such as *Consumer Reports* and *Consumer Digest*, I compiled the information in Tips 495 through 500:

495. *Cross-country ski machines.* The trick to using a cross-country ski machine effectively is to shift your weight from the ball of one foot to the ball of the other foot as your feet glide forward and backward. If you don't shift your weight, you'll just end up shuffling back and forth. It's helpful at the start not to use the arm mechanism at all. Just focus on your feet. It's permissible to even stare at your feet at first. Once you master the rhythm of the movement, however, you should always look up so that you have

good posture and don't get dizzy. Once you're comfortable with your feet, you can add the arm mechanism for extra intensity and upper-body toning. If you don't feel as if you're using your machine correctly, then go visit the store where you purchased it, and don't leave until the salesperson has shown you how to use your machine properly. My favorite was the NordicTrack Pro, which retails for around $600.

496. *Treadmills.* If you would rather not walk in the rain, in dangerous neighborhoods, or in the dark, then a treadmill may be the solution. My favorite was the Pacemaster Six-Pro Soft Step, which retails for around $1,795. Its flexible running deck is great.

497. *Stationary cycle.* As with a treadmill, a stationary cycle can be helpful during the winter and at other times when it's difficult to get outside to cycle. My favorite was the Precor M8.2 E/L cycle trainer, which retails for around $1,200.

498. *Stair climbing machines.* Stair climbing machines offer an intense workout. Be sure to check with your doctor before trying one because stair climbing causes a rapid rise in blood pressure. Leaning forward on the handrails is the most common mistake with using these machines. Leaning reduces the intensity of your aerobic workout by placing too much stress on your back and shoulders. My favorite was the Precor 721E, which retails for around $330.

499. *Rowing.* Rowing is a great full-body workout and is fairly easy to learn. The most important point to remember is to use your full range of motion. Always go all the way forward and backward and move your arms as fully as possible. My favorite was the Nordic-Sport Rower, which retails for around $800.

500. *Weight training.* Free weights (circular weights and bars not connected to a machine) and a simple sturdy bench press that can be converted into an incline bench press work best for weight training. You can often find this equipment at garage sales. Free weights

allow for more natural movements and work a larger number of muscles than weights in machines. Accidents with free weights can cause serious injuries, however. Beginners should seek training from a knowledgeable person and should always work out with an experienced spotter. Of course, the one exercise you can't do with free weights is leg presses. Since you probably want to work out aerobically using your legs at an activity such as running, walking, skiing, or cycling, this usually isn't a problem. Your legs receive a workout while you perform your aerobic exercise. Your upper body receives a workout with free weights.

Everyday Fitness Activities

501. **Shop at garage sales aerobically.** Liven up your usual walking routine by combining it with bargain finding at garage sales. Make arrangements for an hour or two of free time early in the day on a weekend so that you have the first opportunity to snatch up the best deals. If possible, arrange to have a friend go with you. Bargain hunting is often more fun with a friend. Also, you're more likely to carry through on your exercise goals with a friend's support. Depending on your mood, of course, sometimes it's also nice to solo. Get a newspaper with listings of garage sales and a good local map, and target the garage sales you want to visit. Target sales in neighborhoods you'd want to walk through. Maybe there's a particular neighborhood with gorgeous homes, or one with a scenic view. Divide the number of locations you want to visit by the total number of minutes you usually walk to arrive at the approximate time you'll walk at each sale. For example, if you usually walk 30 minutes and you plan to visit three locations, you will walk for 10 minutes at each location. Of course, if some of the locations offer much better walks, then you can spend more time at them. You may want to skip walking at the earlier sales so that you don't miss any bargains. Ideally you want to hit the sales with the best items and worst walking conditions (because you won't be walking) first. Most important, have fun. Make your walks an

adventure. Explore new neighborhoods, talk about your bargains, and when it's all over go out for a chat over a nice hot or cold drink.

502. **Take learning walks.** Develop an interest in something that requires walking to learn and explore. Learn about birds and start walking to watch birds. Learn about geology and start taking walks to explore local geology. Learn about architecture and tour your downtown and neighborhoods to observe local architecture. Learn about plants, flowers, or animals and take walks to observe them. Learn about insects and search your backyard and other areas to collect them. Learn about your local history from ancient times to the present and take walks to observe areas that have historic value for you. Or go to your public library for more ideas. You'll open up new worlds of understanding for yourself and others around you and get a good workout in the process.

503. **Learn everything you can about walking and walk often.** Walking is simple and fun. It clears your mind, it lowers your blood pressure and heart rate, it burns fat, and it's a chance to get in touch with nature and friends. Tips 504 through 509 address the biggest concerns about walking:

504. *Walking and injuries.* While the benefits of walking far outweigh the risks, and while walking is one of the most injury-free forms of exercise available, walking injuries do occur. Plantar fascitis (inflammation of connective tissue in the foot's sole) and heel pain are the most common. To minimize your chances of injury, gradually increase the amount of time and pace you walk, and don't push yourself if something hurts. Also, remember that the biomechanics of running differ from those of walking. Make sure you have a pair of quality walking shoes. Unlike a runner, a walker invariably lands more on the heel and slowly rolls the weight forward to the balls of the feet. Look for the following features in a walking shoe:

- A comfortable padded heel collar, to avoid heel irritation.
- Entire sole designed to absorb shock.
- Bottom of the heel made of carbon rubber or some other long-lasting material.
- Substantial arch supports.
- A toe area with plenty of space allowing your toes ample room to move. Your toes should not be tight against any part of the shoe.
- Uppers made of a high-quality and breathable material such as leather.
- A well-cushioned and supported heel that's slightly higher than the rest of the foot.
- The kind of sole with a rocker profile that enhances a smooth heel-to-toe motion.
- A snug, secure, and comfortable heel.

505. *The right way to walk.* It's important that you walk properly because it's safer, faster, and more rewarding than walking incorrectly. The key is posture. You should not look down at your feet or slump. Over time this can result in chronic lower-back problems. It can also produce instability, as well as tire you out quickly. To build good posture, look straight ahead and see the sky, buildings, trees, and faces of other people when you walk. Your stomach and buttocks should be pulled in and your back straight.

506. *Dogs and walking.* As usual, you'll slither out of bed feeling terrible and not wanting to go for a walk. But then you'll look over at the door and see the dog waiting, shaking with excitement! Just looking at her, and seeing how much she enjoys walking with you, will inspire you to drag yourself from bed and go for a walk. If you have trouble motivating yourself to walk, then you might want to consider acquiring a dog. Dogs are so full of energy and enthusiasm for living that you won't be able to miss a day of walking. Your dog won't let you! Getting a dog also has personal-safety implications. Certain areas where you live may be unsafe to walk

after dark. With a dog at your side and some repellent spray in your fanny pack, you'll be prepared to deter an assailant.

507. *Getting a more intense workout for the same amount of time.* Walk in the snow, on sand, on grass, or over rough terrain. These kinds of surface areas create more walking resistance. As long as you don't slow down, this means you'll get a more intense work-out for the same amount of time spent walking. Of course you can also intensify your workout by walking up hills.

508. *Want even more information?* Write to the Cooper Institute for Aerobics Research and request their *Walking Handbook*. It costs $6.00 including postage. Mail to: Walking Handbook, The Cooper Institute for Aerobics Research, 12330 Preston Road, Dallas, TX 75230, or call (800) 635-7050. You can also write the Rockport Walking Institute for quality educational materials. Their address is: Rockport Walking Institute, P.O. Box 480, Marlboro, MA 01752, or call (508) 485-2090 ext. 114. Information on walking clubs is located in Tips 666 through 668.

509. *Work out and help others by joining various marches such as the March of Dimes' annual WalkAmerica fund-raiser, usually held in late April.* The walk is held in more than 1,450 communities nationwide and is the largest fund-raising event in the United States. All proceeds are used for prevention of birth defects and reduction of infant mortality. For more information, contact your local March of Dimes chapter.

510. **Take the stairs.** Stairs are everywhere. They're in our homes, at work, and in stores. When you combine the availability of stairs with the fact that climbing stairs is a great workout, the result is a truly awesome source of help for any weight-control effort. And yet, few people take the stairs consistently. In a well-known University of Pennsylvania study of 40,000 people, only about 1 percent of overweight people climbed stairs, and only about 5 percent of people in general climbed stairs in a shopping mall, commuter train station, and bus terminal. This is unfortunate because stair

climbing not only is a good workout, but also strengthens your heart and lengthens your life span. Research at Stanford University has shown that, if you climb just 50 steps a day, you'll reduce your risk of heart attack and live longer than if you don't. Climbing stairs is a very intense form of exercise, so check with your health-care professional before getting serious about stairs. In the beginning, also take some time to list opportunities you have during the day to take the stairs. Review your list weekly, add to it, and make sure you're climbing stairs at every opportunity. Tips 511 through 519 contain some ideas to get you started:

511. *Get up from your desk at least every hour to walk up several flights of stairs for a drink of water or to use the bathroom.* You'll usually make up for the few minutes away from your desk by working more efficiently when you return.

512. *Use the upstairs or downstairs bathroom at home.*

513. *If you work or live in a high building, then take the elevator part way up, and climb stairs the rest of the way.*

514. *After an event at a stadium, have a stair-climbing party instead of a tailgate party.*

515. *Form a stair-climbing club and search out unique stairs to climb.*

516. *Try to park your car at the lowest level of a building so that you have to climb stairs to reach your floor.*

517. *At home, place all your telephones upstairs so that you have to climb the stairs to answer the phone.*

518. *Climb up a fairly steep hill near home in the early morning or evening, and enjoy a beautiful sunrise or sunset.*

519. *Go snow sledding or backcountry skiing.* Climbing up the hill or mountain will give you a great workout.

520. **Don't sit still.** Roll your fingers across your desk, tap your toes, squirm around in your chair, pace back and forth when you're on

the phone, or twirl around in your chair. (Try not to annoy any-one.) In the process you'll burn as many as 800 calories in a sin-gle day. That's equivalent to jogging for several miles!

521. **Make your cycling more comfortable.** Stand and pedal 1 minute out of 15 (less often if you're cycling a lot, more often if you're just a beginner). While still out of the saddle, coast and move your hips forward, arching your back. Now sit down and finish by doing several slow neck rolls and shoulder shrugs. You can also vary your hand position every few minutes to reduce your upper-body fatigue.

522. **Commute to work on your bicycle.** Cycling to work is wonderful for your mind, your body, and the environment. You arrive to work feeling clear-headed and invigorated. Unfortunately, many people believe they can't cycle to work for one reason or another. Use Tips 523 through 530 to help you overcome any problems you may have with commuting on your bicycle:

523. *There's no safe place I can park my bike.* Most buildings have out-of-the-way locations you can use. Ask a janitor. If none are avail-able, then try locking your bike to a permanent object such as the bottom of a metal sign, or try storing it with a friendly coworker who lives only a few blocks from work.

524. *I would have to wake up too early if I tried commuting by bike.* You'd be surprised how quickly you can cycle to work. Time your-self in your car and include the time it takes to warm up your car, keep it fueled, and park it. The difference, especially when traffic is heavy, could be much less than you think. In addition, there's the benefit of arriving to work refreshed and alert.

525. *My commute is too far to ride.* Drive to a point that's close enough to allow you to ride your bike the rest of the way, or vice versa.

526. *I need my car for work.* Plan ahead, and on days when you don't need the car take your bike.

527. *I live too close to work.* Take the long way to work.

528. *I don't want to cycle in rush-hour traffic.* There are usually numerous routes you can take to avoid traffic. Get a good street map and plan out a route with small traffic flows. You could also join a health club located nearby. Work out at the club before and after work so that you end up cycling before morning, and after evening, rush hour.

529. *I don't want to ruin my nice clothing.* Leave a week's worth of clothing at work and take your car or public transportation on Monday and Friday.

530. *I don't like riding my bike in poor weather.* Who says you have to ride your bike every day once you start to commute? If the weather is bad, take the car.

531. **Try yoga.** If the thought of yoga fills your head with images of thin people putting their thin legs over their heads and twisting themselves into painful pretzel-like shapes, then you're in for a surprise. When you arrive for your first class, you'll simply find a room full of average people. People dress similarly to what you'd find in an aerobics class, wearing leotards and sweatsuits. Basically, what you do is relax and work out through a combination of deep breathing, concentration, stretching, and strengthening for roughly 60 to 90 minutes. You exercise completely, working even your toes, fingers, eyes, and other small muscle groups. When finished you feel relaxed, strong, confident, and refreshed. You don't get an aerobic fat-burning workout, but the incredible stress relief, combined with the strength and body awareness that yoga promotes, should help your weight-control effort. Yoga classes can be found in the yellow pages under "Yoga." You may also want to try a good video called *Yoga Mind and Body* with Ali MacGraw.

532. **Garden for mind and body.** There's something deeply fulfilling about growing things. Growing plants is creative and a good activity when you feel depressed. Even if it's raining out, you can still go to the garden. A soft, gentle rain can be as uplifting as a bright, sunny sky. In the garden you'll work with your hands in the soil and see right in front of you the results of your labor. You'll feel close to nature, and revived from the fresh air and physical exertion. And don't think gardening isn't a serious workout. Gardening (weeding, spading, digging, and hoeing) one hour is equivalent to walking vigorously at 4 mph for the same amount of time! To get started, go to the library, purchase a gardening book, or subscribe to a quality gardening magazine such as *Organic Gardening* published by Rodale Press, or request information from the National Gardening Association, 180 Flynn Avenue, Burlington, VT 05401.

533. Transform your everyday household chores into fun aerobic workouts. Too many mundane chores to get any exercise? Try turning your cleaning into a workout. Dancing works particularly well. When cleaning and working out, however, it's best not to do any particular dance routine. Rather, just enjoy the music and move to it in whatever way your body wants to express itself. Make an effort to use your entire body. Twist, turn, move your arms, and just let your body flow. Here's a quick-reference list that shows how many calories a 150-pound person burns performing various domestic tasks for one hour:

Baking	137
Washing dishes by hand	135
Washing dishes with dishwasher	110
Making dinner	135
Cleaning windows	210–250
Making beds	210–240
Ironing	205
Scrubbing floors	250–400
Mowing lawn (push power mower)	270
Machine washing and drying clothes	160
Washing and polishing car	230

Shopping	165
Sewing	95
Knitting	95

These figures simply illustrate that these activities are helpful for weight control. Now if you add to these totals the additional 250 calories you'll burn dancing while you clean, you end up with a large calorie burn equivalent to activities such as skipping rope or downhill skiing for an hour! To intensify your workout, try walking up and down stairs a few extra times, jogging in place, or doing step aerobics. Exciting music is the key to a fun cleaning workout. Take some time to put together a collection of music you find motivating. If you have young children, after a while your kids will probably start begging you to clean your home. They'll start to associate house cleaning with playing and will look forward to when mommy puts on the music and dances around the house! There's even a video on exercise and cleaning that contains some tips you may find useful. It's by Victoria Johnson and is called *Clean, Shine and Shape-Up.*

534. **Pop bubbles.** Most people want their weight-control activities to be as fun as possible. If they're fun, you're more likely to perform them often. Well, here's just such an activity. It's called aerobic bubble popping, and it's pure fat-burning fun. When starting, if you want to make your own bubble mixture, buy the Klutz Press book entitled *The Unbelievable Bubble Book.* It comes with a giant bubble wand and contains a good recipe for bubble mixture. It also tells you everything you could ever want to know about bubbles. If you don't want to make your own bubbles, then just go to the store and buy some bubble soap. It's cheap. After you have your soap, take your kids or some friends, go to a big grass playing field that's at least 50 yards long, and check the wind direction. Launch your bubbles upwind of the field so that the wind will blow them across the field. Blow lots of small bubbles, and then just run around and see how many you can pop. See who can

pop the most. After they're all popped, run to the end of the field and then back to your starting location. This will give you more of an aerobic workout. For scores more fun and wacky workouts that can be done with friends or family, see Tips 680 to 727.

535. **Try ballroom dancing.** Once you learn some basic steps, you can dance for extended periods of time and receive a great aerobic workout. What more could a person want? You tone your muscles, you burn up fat, and you enjoy the company of a partner holding you closely! You should begin with classes in swing and foxtrot. These will serve as good building blocks for more difficult dances. Also good at the beginning are classes in Latin dance that teach the rumba, American tango, cha-cha, and mambo. Latin is a favorite of many beginners. You can't miss that strong Latin beat, and it's so enticing and sexy. As with a health club, a dance studio will have special introductory offers. Take advantage of them to check out the activity before committing for the long term. Look for a studio that offers classes that are small for individual attention, well organized, and with enough space to dance comfortably. Also, the instructor should start off each session with a short review of the previous session, since you build the complexity of your dances from week to week. Sometimes community colleges or community centers also will offer quality instruction. There are many ballroom dancing clubs around the country you might want to join. Check your yellow pages, talk with people at dance studios, and locate the club nearest you. Whatever you do, don't say, "Oh, I'm too much of a klutz to try ballroom dancing." Anyone can learn to ballroom dance, and you'll have fun doing it.

536. **Try the new aerobics.** If you haven't been to an aerobics class lately, you might be surprised. The rooms are warmly decorated and inviting, the instructors have skill and extensive training, and the routines are fun. Today you can also select your level of activity, according to your health and fitness level, by choosing from high-impact (both feet off the ground sometimes), low-impact

(one foot on the ground at all times), or no-impact (both feet on the ground at all times) aerobics. If you have low-back, neck, or knee problems, you should avoid floor exercises such as aerobics. If you don't have these problems, however, then the new aerobics may be just what you're looking for. Classes exist for almost every kind of person and every interest. There are classes for seniors, children, new mothers, and even pregnant women. There are classes with jazz, rock, blues, and classical music. There are classes with step benches, weight training, and stretching. There are even aerobics classes for mothers *and* their babies! If you haven't been to an aerobics class lately, check out several of them. When you research a class, look for the following characteristics in your instructor:

- Screens students for health problems and, when needed, provides medical referrals. Screens to make sure students have appropriate clothing and footwear, and directs new students to the appropriate class level.
- Illustrates how to find pulse and target heart-rate range.
- Is certified with a national organization such as the ACSM or AFAA and also maintains updated CPR certification.
- Teaches in a noncompetitive manner and with sincere concern for students.
- Plays music at a volume that doesn't interfere with cues, and uses easy-to-understand cues for transitions.
- Is a good leader and understands proper class format.

537. **Swim away sore joints.** Swimming in open water in a lake or laps in a pool is a wonderful way to receive an aerobic workout and tone muscles without jarring your joints. You must remember when starting, however, that swimming is a *skill*. At the beginning, it's crucial that you get professional instruction. Enroll in a swim class to learn how to crawl stroke, flip turn, and breathe comfortably on both sides. Once you've learned to swim properly,

you'll have a wonderful activity in which you'll be able to participate for life.

Fitness Videos

538. Try an aerobics video. If you prefer to try aerobics at home then
read the exercise-video guide in Tips 539 through 593, or send
your name and address to Video Exercise Catalog, Dept. EF2,
5390 Main Street NE, Minneapolis, MN 55421, and request a free
one-year subscription to *The Complete Guide to Exercise Videos.*
Both of these exercise-video guides will help you choose a video
you will enjoy.

539. Try one of these quality fitness videos. I sifted through more than
2,000 exercise videos to put together this small list of the very best.
All of these videos have excellent cuing, instruction, and transitions and are exciting to view. The guide is divided into beginner,
intermediate, and advanced categories. A beginner is someone
who hasn't exercised consistently in six or more months. An intermediate is someone who is fairly active in some kind of exercise
program two or three times per week. An advanced person is
someone who has been exercising four or more times per week for
at least six consecutive months. Titles are listed alphabetically
within each category.

Beginner

540. *Buns of Steel Startin' Simple Series;* 3 volumes.

541. *Denise Austin's TrimWalk:* Indoor Version.

542. *Gilad's New Beginner Workout.*

543. *Mtv's The Grind Hip Hop Workout.*

544. *Simply Jazzercise with Judi Sheppard Missett;* requires one- to
eight-pound dumbbells.

545. *Susan Powter's Burn Fat and Get Fit;* requires one- to five-pound dumbbells and step.

546. *Tony Little's Cardio Ab Training.*

547. *Tony Little's Cardio Hips, Thighs, and Buns Training.*

548. *Weight Watcher's Easy Shape-Up Healthy Back and Waist Workout.*

549. *Weight Watcher's Easy Shape-Up Lower Body Workout.*

550. *Weight Watcher's Easy Shape-Up Upper Body Workout.*

Intermediate

551. *Basic Training with Ada Janklowicz.*

552. *Brenda Dykgraaf's Combined Whole Body Workout.*

553. *Brenda Dykgraaf's Disco Workout.*

554. *Daisy Fuentes Totally Fit;* requires three- to five-pound dumbbells.

555. *Donna Richardson's Back to Basics.*

556. *Donna Richardson's Step and Awesome Abs;* requires step.

557. *ESPN Fitness Pros—Hip Hop.*

558. *The Firm, Vol. I, Body Sculpting Basics.*

559. *The Firm, Vol. II, Low Impact Aerobics.*

560. *The Firm, Vol. III, Aerobic Interval Training;* requires step.

561. *Gilad's New Best of Bodies in Motion.*

562. *Jane Fonda's Step Aerobic and Ab Workout;* requires step.

563. *Jazzercise Circuit Training;* X-ertube included, requires three- to ten-pound dumbbells and step.

564. *Jodi Cohen's Fitness Country Step Aerobics;* requires step.

565. *Karen Voight's Strong and Smooth Moves;* requires three- to ten-pound dumbbells.

566. *Kari Anderson's Fitness Formula;* requires step.

567. *Kari Anderson's Bench Works;* includes Dynaband and requires step.

568. *Kathy Smith's Great Buns and Thigh Step;* requires step.

569. *Kathy Smith's Step Workout;* requires one- to five-pound dumbbells and step.

570. *Kelly Roberts Real Fitness: Circuit Training;* tape uses a Power-FLEX band, but you can do similar movements with light dumbbells; requires step.

571. *Lynne Brick's Power Stepping II;* requires step.

572. *Nike's Total Body Conditioning;* includes X-ertube; requires three- to five-pound dumbbells and step.

573. *One on One Circuit Training with Gin Miller;* requires five- to eight-pound dumbbells.

574. *Paula Abdul's Get Up and Dance.*

575. *Reebok: The Video with Gin Miller;* requires step.

576. *Slide Reebok Basic Training Workout;* requires slide.

577. *Step Class in a Flash;* requires step.

578. *Tamilee Webb's Building Tighter Assets;* requires one-to five-pound dumbbells and step.

579. *Your Personal Best with Elle Macpherson;* requires one- to five-pound dumbbells.

580. *Victoria Power Shaping II;* requires one- to five-pound dumbbells.

Advanced

581. *Advanced Sliderobics;* requires slide.

582. *Cathe Friedrich's Step Heat;* requires step.

583. *Cia Dynamix 6001 with Lynne Brick;* tape uses a Body Bar (padded 48-inch bar weighing 12 or 18 pounds), but you can substitute dumbbells; requires step.

584. *Creative Instructors Aerobics 4004.*

585. *The Firm Parts: Tough Aerobics;* requires step.

586. *Gilad's Step Aerobics;* requires step.

587. *Gilad's Step and Tone Workout;* requires one- to seven-pound dumbbells and step.

588. *Gin Miller's New Body Workout;* requires three- to five-pound dumbbells.

589. *Karen Voight's Energy Sprint Workout;* requires two- to eight-pound dumbbells and step.

590. *Keli Roberts Real Fitness: Ultimate Step;* requires step.

591. *Reebok Step Circuit Challenge;* requires three- to five-pound dumbbells and step.

592. *Sleek Physique with Barry Joyce;* requires three- to eight-pound dumbbells.

593. *Victoria Johnson's Step with Style;* requires one- to seven-pound dumbbells and step.

Activity Directory

594. **Use this never-get-bored activity directory.** Tips 595 through 671 are a directory of practically every fitness activity that exists. If

one of the activities sounds interesting, then write to the organization and ask them to send you some general information:

595. *Archery:* American Archery Council, 604 Forest Ave., Park Rapids, MN 56470.

596. *Badminton:* United States Badminton Association, 1 Olympic Plaza, Colorado Springs, CO 80909.

597. *Baseball:* National Amateur Baseball Federation, P.O. Box 705, Bowie, MD 20718. See Tips 656 and 657 for information on softball.

598. *Basketball:* Look in the yellow pages under the heading "Basketball Clubs." If none appear, call your local YMCA or check with your park district about clubs, clinics, and pick-up games in your area.

599. *Baton Twirling:* National Baton Twirling Association, Box 266, Janesville, WI 53545.

600. *Bobsled:* U.S. Bobsled and Skeleton Federation, Box 828, Lake Placid, NY 12946. See Tip 628 for information on luge.

601. *Boomerang:* United States Boomerang Association, P.O. Box 182, Delaware, OH 43015.

602. *Bowling:* Your local bowling center is your best source of information.

603. *Curling:* United States Curling Association, c/o David Garber, 1100 Cuter Point Dr., Box 866, Stevens Point, WI 54481.

604. *Cycling:* American Bicycle Association, P.O. Box 718, Chandler, AZ 85244.

605. *Disc Sport:* Ultimate Players Association, 3595 E. Fountain Blvd., Ste. J2, Colorado Springs, CO 80910.

606. *Falconry:* North American Falconer's Association, 820 Jay Pl., Berthoud, CO 80513.

607. *Fencing:* United States Fencing Association, 1750 E. Boulder St., Colorado Springs, CO 80909.

608. *Field Hockey:* United States Field Hockey Association, 1 Olympic Plaza, Colorado Springs, CO 80909.

609. *Fishing:* Bass Anglers Sportsman Society, P.O. Box 17900, Montgomery, AL 36141.

610. *Fishing:* Federation of Fly Fishers, P.O. Box 1519, Bozeman, MT 59771.

611. *Footbag:* World Footbag (HackySack) Association, 1317 Washington Ave., Ste. 7, Golden, CO 80401.

612. *Football:* U.S. Flag and Touch Football League, 7709 Ohio St., Mentor, OH 44060.

613. *Golf:* Your local courses are your best sources of information.

614. *Gymnastics:* USA Gymnastics, 201 S. Capitol, Ste. 300, Indianapolis, IN 46225.

615. *Hiking and Camping:* American Hiking Association, P.O. Box 20160, Washington, DC 20041-2160.

616. *Hiking and Camping:* National Campers and Hikers Association, 4804 Transit Rd. Bldg. 2, Depew, NY 14043.

617. *Hiking and Camping:* Woodswomen, 25 W. Diamond Lake Rd., Minneapolis, MN 55419.

618. *Hockey:* USA Hockey, 4965 N. 30th St., Colorado Springs, CO 80919.

619. *Horse Carriage Driving:* American Driving Society, P.O. Box 160, Metamora, MI 48455.

620. *Horse Trotting:* U.S. Trotting Association, 750 Michigan Ave., Columbus, OH 43215.

621. *Horseshoes:* National Horseshoe Pitchers Association of America, c/o Donnie Roberts, Box 7927, Columbus, OH 43207.

622. *Jai Alai:* U.S. Amateur Jai Alai Players Association, c/o Howard Kalik, 1935 N.E. 150th St., N. Miami, FL 33181.

623. *Jousting:* National Jousting Association, c/o Sandy Izer, P.O. Box 14, Mount Solon, VA 22843.

624. *Juggling:* International Juggler's Association, P.O. Box 218, Montague, MA 01351.

625. *Jump Rope:* American Double Dutch League, P.O. Box 776, Bronx, NY 10451.

626. *Kite Flying:* American Kitefliers Association, 1559 Rockville Pike, Rockville, MD 20852-1651.

627. *Lacrosse:* U.S. Women's Lacrosse Association (USWLA), 35 Wisconsin Circle, Chevy Chase, MD, 20815-7015. The Lacrosse Foundation, 113 W. University Pkwy., Baltimore, MD 21210-3300.

628. *Luge:* U.S. Luge Association, P.O. Box 651, 35 Church St., Lake Placid, NY 12946.

629. *Martial Arts:* National Women's Martial Arts Federation, P.O. Box 4688, Corpus Christi, TX 78469-4688.

630. *Martial Arts:* American Judo Association, 19 N. Union Blvd., Colorado Springs, CO 80909.

631. *Martial Arts:* U.S.A. Karate Federation, 1300 Kenmore Blvd., Akron, OH 44314.

632. *Martial Arts:* U.S. Aikido Federation, 98 State St., North Hampton, MA 01060.

633. *Martial Arts:* U.S. Taikwondo Union, 1750 E. Boulder St., Ste. 405, Colorado Springs, CO 80909.

634. *Motorcycle Riding:* Alliance of Women Bikers, P.O. Box 484, Eau Claire, WI 54702.

635. *Motorcycle Riding:* American Motorcycle Association, P.O. Box 6114, Westerville, OH 43081.

636. *Orienteering:* U.S. Orienteering Federation, P.O. Box 1444, Forest Park, GA 30051.

637. *Paddle Tennis:* United States Paddle Tennis Association, 189 Seeley St., Brooklyn, NY 11218.

638. *Parachuting:* U.S. Parachute Association, 1440 Duke St., Alexandria, VA 22314.

639. *Petanque (outdoor bowling game):* Federation of Petanque USA, c/o Robert E. Morrison, 208 N. Royal St., Alexandria, VA 22314.

640. *Polo on Bicycles:* World Bicycle Polo Federation, P.O. Box 1039, Bailey, CO 80421.

641. *Pool Playing:* American Pool Players Association, 1000 Lake St., St. Louis Blvd., Ste. 325, St. Louis, MO 63367.

642. *Powerlifting:* U.S. Powerlifting Federation, P.O. Box 389, Roy, UT 84067.

643. *Race Carts:* International Kart Federation, 4650 Arrow Hwy., Ste. B4, Montclair, CA 91163.

644. *Racquetball:* American Amateur Racquetball Association, 815 N. Weber, Ste. 101, Colorado Springs, CO 80903.

645. *Rafting, Canoeing, Kayaking:* American Canoe Association, 7432 Alban Station Rd., Ste. B-226, Springfield, VA 22150.

646. *Rafting, Canoeing, Kayaking:* American Whitewater Affiliation, P.O. Box 85, Phoenicia, NY 12464.

647. *Roller-skating:* Artistic Rollerskating Federation, P.O. Box 6579, Lincoln, NE 68506.

648. *Roller-skating:* United States Amateur Confederation of Roller Skating, P.O. Box 6579, Lincoln, NE 68506.

649. *Rowing:* U.S. Rowing Association, 201 S. Capitol Ave., Ste. 400, Indianapolis, IN 46225.

650. *Running:* American Running and Fitness Association, 9310 Old Georgetown Rd., Bethesda, MD 20814.

651. *Sailing:* American Sailing Association, 13922 Marquesas Way, Marina Del Rey, CA 90292.

652. *Shuffleboard:* National Shuffleboard Association, c/o Harold Edmondson, 704 52nd Ave. Dr. W., Bradenton, FL 38207.

653. *Snorkeling, Scuba, and Skin Diving:* Underwater Society of America, P.O. Box 628, Paly City, CA 94017.

654. *Snow Skiing:* American Ski Association, P.O. Box 480067, Denver, CO 80248.

655. *Soccer:* U.S. Soccer Federation, 1801-1811 S. Prairie Ave., Chicago, IL 60616.

656. *Softball:* Amateur Softball Association/National Softball Hall of Fame, 2801 N.E. 50th St., Oklahoma City, OK 73111.

657. *Softball:* U.S. Slowpitch Softball Association, 3935 S. Crater Rd., Petersburg, VA 23805.

658. *Speedskating on Ice:* Amateur Speedskating Association, 1033 Shady Lane, Glen Ellyn, IL 60137.

659. *Surfing:* Women's International Surfing Association, 30202 Silver Spur Rd., P.O. Box 512, San Juan Capistrano, CA 92693. Also, check with your local surf shop for information.

660. *Swimming:* U.S. Masters Swimming, 2 Peters Ave., Rutland, MA 01543.

661. *Synchronized Swimming:* U.S. Synchronized Swimming, Pan American Plaza, 201 S. Capitol, Ste. 510, Indianapolis, IN 46225.

662. *Table Tennis:* U.S. Table Tennis Association, 1750 E. Boulder St., Olympic Complex, Colorado Springs, CO 80909.

663. *Tennis:* U.S. Tennis Association, 1217 Ave. of the Americas, New York, NY 10036.

664. *Triathlons:* Triathlon Federation, 3595 E. Fountain Blvd., Colorado Springs, CO 80910.

665. *Volleyball:* U.S. Volleyball Association, 3595 E. Fountain Blvd., Colorado Springs, CO 80910-1740.

666. *Walking:* American Volksport Association, Phoenix Sq., 1001 Pat Booker Rd., Ste. 203, Universal City, TX 78148.

667. *Walking:* National Organization of Mall Walkers, P.O. Box 191, Herman, MO 65041.

668. *Walking:* Walkabout International, 835 Fifth Ave., Room 407, San Diego, CA 92101.

669. *Water Polo:* 201 S. Capitol, Ste. 520, Indianapolis, IN 46225.

670. *Water Skiing:* American Water Skiing Association, 799 Overlook Dr., Winterhaven, FL 33884.

671. *Wrestling:* U.S.A. Wrestling, 225 S. Academy Blvd., Colorado Springs, CO 80910.

10.

Tips on Coping with Family

672. Make certain your mate isn't keeping you fat. Sometimes the person you love most can be your biggest weight-control obstacle. For myriad reasons, most of which stem from insecurity, some people do everything they can to keep their mates fat. Sometimes their strategies are subtle and difficult to recognize but still effective. To help you identify these kinds of strategies, and increase your awareness of this phenomenon, Tips 673 through 679 list some strategies people might use to keep their mates fat:

673. *Mates may demand irresistible foods.* For instance, George knows that his wife can't resist her own famous chocolate chip brownies. So George begins to complain that she should make brownies "for the children." His wife begins to feel guilty about not baking as much for her family, and starts making brownies again "for the children." As in the past, she eats most of them before the children come home from school.

674. *Mates may tempt or reward with high-calorie snacks.* They tempt their spouses by eating their favorite fatty and sugary snacks in front of them and constantly offering to share with them. Mates also might reward their spouses with high-calorie snacks for achieving a weight-loss goal.

675. *Mates may practice grocery undermining.* They may offer to do the grocery shopping and then come home with fatty foods.

676. *Mates may demoralize.* "Who are you kidding? You've always failed before and will fail again."

677. *Mates may complain about money.* Mates complain about every little thing that costs extra as a result of their mate's weight control such as memberships, clothing, classes, or equipment.

678. *Mates may complain about loneliness.* Mates complain about how lonely they feel when their mate leaves the house to exercise, even if it's for just 30 minutes!

679. *1,000 dirty deeds.* Mates may become very demanding just before their mate wants to exercise. For instance, it's almost too dark to run, Jane has on her running clothes, has just fed and bathed the kids and washed the dishes, and is about to go out the door when she hears her husband yell, "Could you please iron my shirts right now; I need them for my big trip tomorrow."

680. **Have a blast burning fat with your family.** It's a fact that after you have children your chances for becoming overweight increase dramatically. Much of this phenomenon results from environmental factors such as increased stress and tension, and no longer having any time for yourself. There's also the guilt that comes from working all day, and then not spending as much time in the evening with your children because you're out exercising. One solution is to find as many activities as possible that you *and* your children enjoy. This strategy allows you to bond with your children in a fun way, gives all of you exercise, and saves money, since you won't need a sitter.

     The best way to get a vigorous walking or running workout with your children before they can run or cycle is with a baby jogger. A baby jogger has three big bicycle wheels and a seat in the middle, and you run or walk behind it. Infant backpacks also work well for going over rough terrain such as you would encounter during a hike. These are available at outdoor stores and work well, especially if your spouse carries it! For cyclists, there are cycling carts you can buy to pull your kids behind your bike. These are much safer than putting an infant seat on the back of your bike, because when the baby rocks back and forth in the infant seat, it can make you unstable.

Tips 681 through 727 describe fun activities to do with older children. Many of the activities are best with two "teams." If you need more people, call up your friends and invite them to come out and play.

681. *Animal aerobics.* When doing animal aerobics with your children, go around and around in a circle about 35 yards wide. Keep moving all the time, and with each lap change to a new animal behavior in Tips 682 to 695. When you're done, walk around slowly to warm down.

682. *Hop like a bunny.*

683. *Crawl like a crocodile.*

684. *Walk like a spider.*

685. *Run and roar like a tiger.*

686. *Fly with your arms flapping up and down like a condor.*

687. *Walk heavily with your arm in front like an elephant.*

688. *Run like a monkey with your hands dragging on the ground.*

689. *Hop like a frog.*

690. *Gallop like a wild horse.*

691. *Run like a bull, using your fingers for horns.*

692. *Run sideways like a sidewinder snake.*

693. *Run backwards like a two-headed dragon.*

694. *Hop like a kangaroo.*

695. *Buzz and fly like a bumblebee.*

696. *Hide and seek.* This is fun with little kids especially. You can do this indoors or outside.

697. *Freeze tag.* Usually it's your spouse and you versus the kids. You divide into two teams with one team being "it" and the other team

"not it." The team that's "it" has to try to touch a member of the team that's "not it." Once touched, you have to freeze until a teammate can sneak up and "unfreeze" you. Once a team is frozen, that game is over and the other team becomes "it." This works best in a place with obstacles to run around.

698. *Frog jumping.* Everyone pretends to be frogs and starts jumping all over the place. The leader frog then cries out commands such as jump side to side, forward and backward, or in place, jump and clap, then jump "all together" to the finish line.

699. *Simon says.* This is a classic and lots of fun. If someone moves after you give a command that doesn't start with "Simon says," the player is out of the game. You stop the activity by saying, "Simon says stop." You can order players to jump, run, skip, swim in the air with their arms, and all sorts of actions that you're also doing with them simultaneously.

700. *Keep away.* You divide into two teams and one team tries to "keep away" a ball or Frisbee from the other.

701. *Follow the leader.* Players go around the field trying to do whatever the leader does. The second person in line goes to the front, and the leader goes to the back, every minute or so.

702. *Dance blasting.* Turn up the volume on your stereo, radio, or whatever and start to dance. Give awards for the craziest dance, the fastest dance, the slowest dance, the silliest dance, and others you create. Make a rule that when the music quits dancers have to freeze just as they are.

703. *Aerobic kite flying.* Toss a kite in the air and use only your running ability to keep it flying. Run down the field flying the kite, then walk back to the start. Then run down the field again, and then walk back to the start again until you've had enough. The kids won't want you to stop and will cheer you on so they can see the kite fly. Don't let them down!

704. *Adventure hikes.* Get a hiking book, plan out a mild hike for kids that will work for you and your children, pack a lunch, and take along some bird, tree, and plant books. Make it an adventure for your kids. You may find it fun to read them an adventure story, and then to pretend you're the people in the story during your hike.

705. *Flatland sled races.* Who says you need a hill to sled? Go to a field and run across it with your kids in the sled. Pretend you're the horse and have them sing "Jingle Bells." Let them pretend to crack a whip if you think you'll need it!

706. *Giant sand and snow sculptures.* Building a sand or snow sculpture is a good muscle workout, fun for the kids, and educational. Don't limit yourself to just sand castles and snowmen—also try fish, cats, dogs, or whatever you're in the mood for.

707. *Cross-country ski sledding.* When your kids are about four to six years of age, try pulling them in a sled behind you while you ski. You don't want to go on steep courses, or the sled may crash into you. Fairly flat beginner courses work well.

708. *Juggling.* Juggling helps you relax, builds coordination, and is a good workout. Kids love it too, especially when combined with music. You can try juggling scarves, plastic bowling pins, rings, fake swords, and all kinds of things.

709. *Frisbee.* Don't just stand around. Be sure to throw the Frisbee so that the other person has to run for it. Running for the Frisbee, and running around acting silly between tosses, will give you more of an aerobic workout.

710. *Roly poly.* Go to the top of a hill, and then roll down it on your side. (Check for dog waste first if necessary.) This is fun in both the summer and winter. After you reach the bottom, run back up to the top and do it again. Don't go too fast down when you're first starting, or you might make yourself sick.

711. *Musical chairs.* Everyone probably knows how to play this. In case you forgot, you have a circle with one fewer chair than the number of people you have. You turn on the music and play it for a while, while everyone walks around the chairs, and then stop it. Everyone scrambles for the chairs, and the person who doesn't get one is out. You then remove one chair and do it again and again until only one person remains in one chair. To turn this into a workout, do it outside and make the circle a big one.

712. *Find it and keep it.* Buy a bunch of cheap toys or water balloons and then hide them all over the place for the kids to find. Time yourself to see how long it takes for you to hide them.

713. *Collecting walks.* Go on walks to collect bugs, rocks, leaves, or whatever. Kids love to collect all kinds of things, and the walking is good for you.

714. *Mall walking.* I'm sure you know about this. A day spent walking around the mall can be quite a workout. Just don't binge on fast food or junk food while shopping. It usually works best to mall walk right after you've eaten, and then to head home before you get hungry.

715. *The course of torment.* It's fun to set up obstacle courses with your kids, and then see who can run through them the fastest. Use chairs, blankets, orange cones, white spray paint on grass, chalk on pavement, whatever you want to use to mark the course and to make it challenging. In winter, make marks in the snow and construct obstacles from snow.

716. *Kick the can.* Place a can out in the middle of a big field; then form two teams. One team guards the can while the other tries to kick it without getting tagged in the process. Once someone is tagged, that person is placed in "prison." The only way for the player to get out of prison is for someone on the prisoner's team to kick the can. If everyone on a team ends up in prison, that team loses. If they kick the can, they win.

717. *Volleyball.* With young children it's fun to use a giant ball and try to hit it as high as you can each time rather than playing real volleyball.

718. *Stress-reducing water fights.* Keep squirt guns and water balloons handy at all times during the summer. When you're ready for some cooling fun, invite your kids outside for a water fight. They'll love it. (Make sure you pick up the balloon pieces—they're a choking hazard.)

719. *Relay races.* Divide into teams of at least two people; then race to a point and back to the beginning to tag the next person to start. When your team has finished, with everyone going three times or whatever, you're done. The first team done wins. The kinds of relays you can create are limited only by your imagination. Tips 720 through 727 describe some favorite relay races:

    720. *Running with an egg on a spoon.*

    721. *Running with a book or something else on your head.*

    722. *Running while trying to kick a ball in front of you.*

    723. *Somersaulting all the way down and back.*

    724. *Hopping.*

    725. *Using a teaspoon to empty the cup of water at the start into the empty cup at the finish.* Points are scored for finishing first, and for transporting the most water without spilling.

    726. *Leapfrogging.* One person leaps as a frog over the person in front of him or her, who's crouched down. Then the person who was just leapt over leaps over the person who just landed in front of him or her. Do this all the way down and back, and then tag the next group of two.

    727. *Water balloon relay.* Each person carries a water balloon. To tag the next person in line, you have to throw the balloon and break it on the next person.

728. **Try not to buy treats for the kids.** Don't kid yourself—as soon as you're in the car you're going to start eating them. Buy for the kids

only when they're with you, and tell them exactly what you bought them. They'll make certain you don't eat their treats.

729. **Avoid eating the kids' leftovers.** The best strategy here is to have the plates cleared and scraped clean immediately after your child has finished eating.

730. **Stop the nagging.** People close to you often think they're doing you a favor by nagging you about your weight. Believe it or not, they think they're helping to motivate you. Most of the time, however, nagging has just the opposite effect. For example, if your spouse is always nagging you to stop eating chocolate ice cream, suddenly chocolate ice cream never tasted so good! If nagging is a problem for you, it's important to make the people around you aware that their nagging isn't helping. Try taking two weeks to record in a diary how many times they nag you about your weight each day, then tactfully confronting them with your written proof.

731. **Try not to get upset when your mate doesn't notice.** Lose weight for you. Don't do it for anybody else, not even your mate. If your mate doesn't notice you've lost 10 pounds, so what? You're doing it for yourself.

732. **Experiment with strategies when your family eats and snacks in front of you.** When you're the only one in your family trying to lose weight, you can feel separated, deprived, alone, and sometimes angry. It may not seem fair they can have what you can't. First communicate to your family that this really bothers you. If talking through the problem doesn't work, then another strategy is to fight taste with taste. Develop as many wonderful low-fat snacks and meals as you can, and then prepare them often so that cooking them becomes second nature. Be realistic when you select your recipes, and focus on simple recipes that are easy to fix. Remember that most people eat only about 10 different recipes all year long. You don't need 200 recipes.

733. **Have lots of sex, and for longer periods of time.** Sex is a very satisfying way to unwind and feel loved. Read books on it, keep an open mind, and increase your level of sexual activity. For starters you might want to read Lori Salkin's and Rob Sperry's *365 Ways to Make Love*, available at bookstores. Most important, remember that as with any exercise, the longer you do it the better for fat burning.

734. **Keep food and love separate.** Many people associate food with love. For instance, your mother may have a way of baking for months prior to your visit, and then loading you up with suitcases full of food when you leave. Take some time to talk about this with your mother. Let her know that hugs, pats on the back, kind words, and sharing experiences are better expressions of love for you than food.

735. **Help your children not to become overweight adults.** This obviously isn't a simple way to lose weight. Nevertheless, it's a very important issue and so I've included it here anyway. While there are no guarantees your child will end up at a healthy weight at maturity, adhering to the following guidelines should help:

736. *Don't give food rewards.* Why do people reward their children with food? It's probably because a food reward is what you were given as a child, and so it's the first thing that pops into your head as an adult. To stop giving food rewards, first involve your kids in the process. Sit down with them to make a list of nonfood rewards they would like, that don't cost very much, and that would be easy for you to give. By having the children help put the list together, you've reduced the possibility they'll whine for candy when you give them the reward they chose. Perhaps more important, you can refer to the list at a glance, and that's just what you need during your busy day.

It's also helpful to create two lists, one for big achievements and the other for smaller achievements. For big achievements, such as an excellent report card, you could buy them a new Lego box or toy accessory, or maybe rent a children's movie. For smaller achievements, such as good behavior at the table, you might read them a favorite bedtime story or let them stay up five minutes longer, have a bubble bath, or play outside five minutes longer.

737. *Don't make your children eat every morsel.* It's okay if they don't finish everything on their plates. Let your kids' natural appetite control express itself. When one of your kids doesn't eat something you think he or she should, take a few deep breaths, relax, and consider whether the child really does need to eat it, or whether you should give in and allow your child to regulate his or her own eating.

738. *Set firm limits.* Children crave discipline. It's an integral part of their development. Kids need limits. But there's no kid anywhere who *needs* a bottle of soda pop or a chocolate candy bar. It's up to you as a parent to set limits and stick to them with consistency. If your kids complain, nag, whine, cry, yell, and even scream, "I hate you!" it's all a part of their complex emotional development. When you set reasonable limits and consistently enforce them, it helps your children learn good eating habits and develop self-control.

739. *Don't use food to become closer with your child.* Don't go buy a pint of gourmet ice cream to share with your child to have an intimate moment. For true intimacy, develop mutual interests. For example, if you and your daughter both like flowers, spend time together going to shops and shows, sharing books and magazines, and working together in the garden.

740. *Have them participate in a sport.* Be sure they understand that gym class isn't representative of what it's like participating in a sport you love. Talk to your children and together discover a sport that *they* would enjoy. Expose them to a number of sports, and then let them decide which ones to pursue. A sport should also help limit your child's television time. It's a fact that people who watch a lot of television are more likely to be overweight than

those who don't. See Tips 886 through 889 for more advice on reducing television time.

741. *Be a good role model.* The most important thing you can do for your child is to have healthy eating and fitness habits yourself. In one remarkable success story, a daughter was so inspired by her mother's success at finally losing her weight and keeping it off, the daughter then lost 100 pounds!

742. **Don't be a grouch—work with your family.** If your weight control makes you grouchy, be careful to control your bad moods and not to direct them toward your family. It's easy to take your family for granted and act like a grouch all the time. (Grouchiness is common at the start of a weight-control program. For more on this, read Tip 942.) Remember, however, that family support can make losing weight much easier, so it's important not to alienate your family from your weight-control effort. To start working with your family, sit down together to discuss whichever of the following guidelines you think might help:

743. *Ask them not to expect perfection.* Make sure they understand that no one is perfect and you're no exception. Tell them it will help you if they don't make a big deal out of setbacks. They're a natural and healthy part of any new process.

744. *Ask for encouragement.* Emphasize to them that you need to be encouraged rather than scolded or lectured when you make a mistake.

745. *Tell them not to hide any treats around the house.* You may find them and feel tempted or resentful.

746. *Ask them to be nice to you.* This will help you maintain a positive attitude, whereas nagging, threats, and coercion will probably make you want to eat more.

747. *Ask the family to develop new interests with you.* Ask them to mirror the new behaviors you're trying to learn. For instance, if you're

trying to slow down your eating by taking time out halfway through your meals with a cup of tea, ask them to join you.

748. *Make specific requests for help.* Don't just say, "I could really use some help." Instead, say, "Will you watch junior for 30 minutes while I go for a walk." Or, "Please clear the table so I don't overeat while I clean up."

749. *Tell your family you love them and that they're most important in your life.* The fact that you have to leave to exercise, or don't bake cookies for them, doesn't mean you love them any less. You will be expressing your love in new ways.

750. *Communicate.* Meet at least once a month to discuss your weight control with your family.

751. *Take responsibility.* Reassure your family that you're only asking for their help, and that you'll take full responsibility for your actions. When you slip up, you won't blame them for being overly critical or not critical enough.

752. *Ask your family to be as relaxed, upbeat, and encouraging as they possibly can.*

753. **Try the team approach when confronting critical in-laws.** Does your mother-in-law gasp when you order dessert, or criticize your cooking, eating, wardrobe, and everything else? If so, a team approach may help. Candidly discuss the situation with your spouse. Together create a team strategy to deal with your mother-in-law. The key is to have your spouse's complete support. It's your spouse's opinion your mother-in-law will listen to. After you've talked, then confront your mother-in-law as a team. Be kind and tactful, but also firm enough that you make yourself clear. With your spouse voicing the concerns that you both wish to address, you have a good chance of eliminating or reducing your mother-in-law's criticism once and for all.

754. **Try not to feel selfish for focusing on yourself.** Doing things for yourself will make the time you do spend with your family that much better.

755. **Share to avoid mealtime competition.** When families sit down to eat they often click into "big family mode" and start to devour as much food as they can as fast as they can. Dinner conversation doesn't exist. One solution to this eating frenzy is to have everyone in your family serve a partner before serving him- or herself. Rotate partners nightly so that competing teams don't form.

756. **Buy holiday candy you hate.** At Halloween, Christmas, Easter, birthdays, and other special days, buy only candy you can't stand to eat. An even better strategy is to give away nickels or cheap toys instead of candy.

757. **Visit family after dinner.** If dinner at your mother's or mother-in-law's house proves too much of a strain for you, then try visiting after dinner.

758. **Consider not eating with the kids.** Enjoy a relaxed atmosphere with your spouse during dinner and have the kids eat someplace else. If you spend lots of time with your kids during the day, then what's wrong with eating alone with your spouse for 30 minutes? You can interact with the kids after dinner. A family doesn't have to eat together to be a close family. You can eat and then enjoy each other without food.

759. **Voice your need for appreciation.** Many people overeat to compensate for what they perceive is a lack of appreciation from family members. The lack of appreciative expressions such as hugs, pats on the back, romance, or expressions of thanks causes many people to bury their disappointment in fatty, sugary food. Communication is the best strategy to avoid overeating because of a lack of appreciation. It's up to you to tell others that you don't feel appreciated, and exactly what they can do to help. Don't just say, "It would be nice to get some appreciation around here." Rather,

to your spouse say something such as, "I would like you to hug me every time you leave for work and as soon as you come home. I would like you to thank me for cooking after every meal, and I would like you to do something special for me a few times a month to show your appreciation (flowers, dancing, hiking, a long romantic walk together). With kids, it's helpful to list all you do for them, and then to post it in the kitchen so that they understand all your hard work. For example, your list could contain some of the following:

- All the rooms you keep clean
- All the meals you make and the planning and shopping involved
- Washing dishes
- Cleaning clothes
- Paying bills
- Earning money
- Driving them around
- Mowing the grass

Do your best to make them understand how much difference it makes to you when they show their appreciation.

11.

Tips on Keeping a Positive Attitude

Getting Motivated

760. **You've gotta get real.** People who start their weight-control effort thinking they can lose lots of weight in a month or so and look beautiful for the rest of their lives are prime targets for scam diet ads that always say things such as "5-Day Miracle Diet," or "Drop 50-Plus Pounds in 30 Days," or "Thin Thighs Like Magic." The solution here is to remember that "fast and easy" and "permanent weight loss" are opposites! They don't go together, and they never will. Once you understand that, you can begin to piece together a real-world weight-control plan that works. You don't think you'll discover 500-year-old gold coins in the basement of your suburban home. Why should you think you can lose 50 pounds in five months and keep it off? Have you ever tried to *lift* 50 pounds? It's a lot of weight! And when you fail to achieve the nearly impossible, what happens? You experience self-doubt, frustration, anger, resignation, depression, and other nasty things. Get real. A reasonable real-world weight loss you could expect to achieve would be around 1 pound per week.

To make losing weight at this rate tangible and therefore motivating, try creating a graph you can call My Realistic Weight-Loss Graph. To make this graph, first assume you'll lose 1 pound per week, and that this will produce a 16-pound weight loss in 16 weeks. Using the graph in Appendix E, you can then draw a line with a straight-edge ruler from the 0 mark on the left, down diagonally to the right, so that your line ends at a point vertically over 16 weeks and horizontally along −16 pounds. Finish by filling in the dates for each week numbered at the bottom. Mark on your personal calendar that you'll check this graph in four weeks. When the four weeks end, check your graph to see how your weight loss is progressing.

As you lose at a realistic rate, keep in mind the many *years* you've probably already wasted failing to lose weight fast and easily. Think of weight control as a Chinese finger puzzle. The harder and faster you try to free your fingers from the puzzle, the more firmly you become entrapped. But if instead you slowly ease your fingers from the puzzle, then gradually you can work them free. The same is true with losing weight. A gradual approach works best. Next time you feel as if you have to rush to achieve a weight-control goal, try saying the following phrase to yourself: "It's because I'm in a hurry that I must go slowly." Commit to a slow and steady weight loss. It's truly the easiest and fastest method for permanent weight control you'll ever find.

761. **Try the six-month rule.** There are two fundamental problems with almost all weight-control programs today. On the one hand, some programs will enable you to lose weight relatively quickly and therefore will motivate you enough to lose weight. The problem with these programs, however, is that they don't give your mind enough time to adjust to your rapidly shrinking body and brand-new lifestyle. Consequently it's almost inevitable you'll gain all your weight back within two years. On the other hand, viable long-term programs that really work typically progress very slowly. Consequently people can't stay motivated enough to continue these realistic programs for more than two or three weeks.

As a solution, you may want to try the six-month rule. Research on more than 4,000 people by the Cooper Institute has revealed that people who exercise aerobically for six consecutive months will likely succeed in making aerobic exercise an enjoyable and fun part of their lives. Research on more than 2,000 women as part of the Women's Health Trial has revealed that many women no longer crave fat, and some women actually lose their taste for fat, after six months on a low-fat diet. Next time you start a weight-control program of exercising more and consuming fewer calories and fat grams, don't make it your goal to lose X number of pounds. Focus instead on achieving and maintaining your exercise and eating goals for six months. In other words, with the six-month rule your overall goal now wouldn't be to lose 30 pounds. Your overall goal would be, for instance, to walk 30 minutes a day and not to exceed your daily calorie and fat-gram goals for six full months. This shift in your overall goal from pounds lost to persevering for six months might be all it takes to keep you from becoming depressed and quitting during the first critical weeks of your program.

762. **Use a fat-attack graph for motivation.** In the past, first you'd get excited about some new diet you thought was really going to work. Then you'd talk about it with friends for a week or two, set a start date, and go for it. Usually you'd start out strong and lose some weight, maybe 10 pounds, and then your weight loss would start to slow way down. Some weeks you'd lose a pound, some weeks you'd gain a pound. It was always the same, and it was at this point that you became depressed and gave up. Sound familiar? Try using the Fat-Attack Graph in Appendix F to motivate you next time your weight loss slows. This graph has the weeks across the bottom, and your weight loss down the left side. To use it, weigh yourself each week and plot your weight change on the graph. As before, you'll gain weight some weeks and lose weight others, but with the graph you'll be able to see visually that overall you're losing. It's also helpful to have a diary to go along with the graph. This helps you better understand why you aren't losing at certain times, and why you are losing at other times.

763. Make a pro/con list to deal with the last 10 pounds. Losing the last 10 pounds can be the most difficult and frustrating part of the weight-loss process. Consequently you may want to ask yourself if you really need to lose those last 10 stubborn pounds. By now you're probably at a healthy weight and you look and feel better than you have in years. Why suffer through 10 more pounds of weight loss to conform to some standard of social beauty? Not everyone has to look like a magazine cover model to be happy. It can be helpful to make a pro/con list. The column against continuing to lose weight should contain things you can be happy about at your present weight, such as:

- You don't have to tear apart your closet hoping to find something that fits.
- No more elastic waistbands.
- You can walk down the street and people don't stare at you.
- You can find your clothing size in most department stores and can choose from a large selection.
- You're at a healthy weight and have done much to reduce your risk for heart disease, cancer, and stroke.
- People think you look pretty good and have congratulated you on the weight you've already lost.
- In-laws and waiters don't look twice when you order dessert.
- You see a much thinner and toned body when you look at yourself in the mirror.
- You're more active now than you've been in years.
- Your self-confidence is high.

   The column for continuing to lose weight should contain compelling reasons for proceeding such as:

- Health concerns
- Self-esteem
- Quality of life
- Personal pride

Writing a pro/con list for this decision will either motivate you to continue or help you to feel happy about stopping where you are now. It's a very personal choice only you can make. Don't let perfect images on women's magazines decide for you, don't let your spouse decide for you, don't let your friends decide for you. It's ultimately up to you.

764. **Get motivated and stay that way.** The key here is to realize that *long-term* motivation is a personal and internal phenomenon. It's not something that someone else can instill in you. Weight control is a lifetime commitment, and no seminar in the world can psyche you up for a lifetime! The motivation has to be internal. You must have a compelling reason why you want to lose weight.

For some this motivation is the result of midlife. They come to realize they can't do anything about growing older but they can do something about controlling their weight to improve the quality of their lives. Others find motivation in health concerns. They've reached a point where they know, if they don't control their weight, they're going to shorten their life spans. For others motivation comes from years of failure. They've tried and tried and failed and failed, and one day they finally get fed up with it all and just do it. For still others it's for purely cosmetic reasons, and that's fine too, as long as you're truly passionate about it. Whatever the reasons, and there are lots of them, all of these motivations have one thing in common. They're all compelling motivations that stir the soul within. They aren't superficial motivations, such as losing for a big vacation, or for your friend's wedding.

Take some time to ask yourself exactly why you want to lose weight, and write out the answers. Once you have a clear understanding of what's motivating you, then you'll be better able to draw on those feelings for strength and support. If it turns out you can't find any compelling reason why you want to lose weight, then you should consider abandoning your weight-control effort until you're more serious.

765. **Use the many dangers of too much fat for motivation.** One glance at the following list of health problems related to being overweight should be enough to motivate anyone who is carrying around too much fat, and wants to live a long and healthy life, to lose weight:

- Breast cancer
- Colon cancer
- Prostate cancer
- Heart attack
- Stroke
- High blood pressure
- Diabetes mellitus
- Surgical complications
- Back pain
- Arthritis
- Hernias
- Hemorrhoids
- Gallbladder disease
- Breathing difficulties
- Hearing loss
- Sleeping disorders

Glance at the Body Mass Index (BMI) in Table 4 to assess your present condition. While this chart doesn't take into account crucial factors such as overall build, percentage body fat, or age, it does show that acceptable weights fall within a range. The acceptable range for most people is a BMI of 20 to 25, but potential health problems increase as your weight increases. If your BMI climbs above 25, you've increased your risk for all of the problems on the preceding list. Don't fool yourself: you're not indestructible. If you're overweight, these nasty things are just as likely to happen to you as they are to anyone else. (In addition to maintaining a healthy BMI, you should make sure your blood pressure is less than 140/90, and that your cholesterol is under 200 mg/dl.)

Table 4

BODY MASS INDEX													
19	20	21	22	23	24	25	26	27	28	29	30	35	40
HEIGHT″						WEIGHT							
58	91	96	100	105	110	115	119	124	129	134	138	143	167	191
59	94	99	104	109	114	119	124	128	133	138	143	148	173	198
60	97	102	107	112	118	123	128	133	138	143	148	153	179	204
61	100	106	111	116	122	127	132	137	143	148	153	158	185	211
62	104	109	115	120	126	131	136	142	147	153	158	164	191	218
63	107	113	118	124	130	135	141	146	152	158	163	159	197	225
64	110	116	122	128	134	140	145	151	157	163	169	174	204	232
65	114	120	126	132	138	144	150	156	162	168	174	180	210	240
66	118	124	130	136	142	148	155	161	167	173	179	186	216	247
67	121	127	134	140	146	153	159	166	172	178	185	191	223	255
68	125	131	138	144	151	158	164	171	177	184	190	197	230	262
69	128	135	142	149	155	162	169	176	182	189	196	203	236	270
70	132	139	146	153	160	167	174	181	188	195	202	207	243	278
71	136	143	150	157	165	172	179	186	193	200	208	215	250	286
72	140	147	154	162	169	177	184	191	199	206	213	221	258	294
73	144	151	159	166	174	182	189	197	204	212	219	227	265	302
74	148	155	163	171	179	186	194	202	210	218	225	233	272	311
75	152	160	168	176	184	192	200	208	216	224	232	240	279	319
76	156	164	172	180	189	197	205	213	221	230	238	246	287	328

766. Lose weight for reasons related to weight control. Losing weight will make you healthier, more energetic, and more confident. These positive factors will snowball into other areas of your life, making you a better person and improving the quality of your life. Losing weight in itself won't, however, magically fix a deteriorating marriage or friendship, help you get along better with your teenage daughter, or produce a wonderful social life. Lose weight for reasons related to weight control such as improved health, appearance, self-confidence, or quality of life, and you'll take a big step toward ensuring you'll be able to keep the weight off once and for all.

767. **Get excited when your weight loss slows.** If you're losing weight rapidly and easily at the very start of your weight-control program, it's probably water loss. This is because your body rids itself of water when your intake of salt and carbohydrate decreases. Two or three weeks into your program you'll start to lose both fat and water and your weight loss will slow. Eventually your body will get down to the hard-core fat. At this point your weight loss will really slow. This is a critical time in your weight-control program. A good way to cope with this potentially frustrating situation is to remember that it's only at this point that you're starting to lose primarily fat! Remember, it's the fat you're after. Weight loss is just an easy way to keep track of fat loss. So don't feel let down when your "weight loss" starts to slow down. This is the time when you should start to become most excited. Through work and commitment you've finally arrived at the point where you can start to purge your body of its excess fat.

768. **Keep a gratitude journal.** There's a common saying that an optimist looks at a glass filled halfway and thinks it's "half full." A pessimist looks at the same glass and thinks it's "half empty." It can be difficult, but be as optimistic as possible about your life so that you reduce stress, depression, and hopelessness. One tool that can help you do this is called a gratitude journal. Purchase a blank bound journal from a bookstore or stationery store. In it, write five things that you're thankful for at the end of each day to reinforce your optimism. While pondering your day, look inward to find happiness in simple everyday occurrences such as good health, abundant healthy food, a warm safe bed, an invigorating walk, a greater sense of control, or a pleasant phone call from a close friend. This will help you end the day on a positive note and look forward to tomorrow.

769. **Create a laugh library.** Develop an arsenal of comedy-filled books and videotapes to read and watch whenever you become depressed, anxious, or frustrated. There's nothing like a good hard laugh to get you back on your feet. Laughing relaxes muscles,

lowers blood pressure, and stimulates production of the same stress-reducing hormones triggered by exercise. When you feel like bingeing, look through your personal laugh library instead, and it's almost inevitable you'll feel better. Once you feel better, you can start to identify the cause of your depression and deal with it.

770. **Don't wait until you've lost your weight to start living.** Yes, you can work on losing weight and really "live" at the same time! Don't put off buying new clothes, trips, social functions, going to the beach, or other fun things until you lose your weight. Get out and do them now. This may seem obvious, but many people can't seem to get past the attitude that they have to punish and deprive themselves in order to lose weight. The fact is, by depriving and punishing yourself, you're actually making it much more likely you won't lose. All deprivation does is set you up for a big fat binge. So don't postpone your life until you've lost your weight. Get out and have fun now.

771. **Make mood swings work for you.** Try channeling your negative energy into exercise. It takes some practice, but what you can do when you hit a low point in your mood cycle is force yourself to get out the door. If you can just get out the door, you'll be on your way to recovery. Once out the door, exercise by either walking, running, or whatever. Through physical activity you'll feel as if you're doing something positive to put your pieces back together. The mood swing will work *for* you when you use all that negative energy for a fat-burning workout.

772. **Visit a pet store when you're depressed.** Watching little kittens and puppies play, wrestle, and tease each other will take your mind off your problems. And the drive and walking to and from the pet store will give you time to identify and cope with your problems without food.

773. **Read weight-control success stories.** Read and reread weight-control success stories for motivation and inspiration. You can find sources for these stories under North American Weight-Control

Survey in the Suggested Readings at the back of this book. These are stories about people who lost weight and kept it off and how they did it. Put together a collection of them and whenever you become depressed or lazy start to read through them. These stories can inject you with confidence and enthusiasm. You may say to yourself, "Hey, if she can do it, so can I." The home videos *Flash Dance* and the original *Rocky* are also excellent for success-story-type motivation.

774. **Try the power of prayer.** You may want to try praying about your weight control. Set small, attainable goals, and then use prayer to help you achieve them. You could also ask family, friends, or church members to pray for you to lose your weight and keep it off. The additional support of many people all praying to help you achieve your goal could be very helpful.

775. **Focus on your positives.** You may be in the habit of standing in front of a mirror and saying to yourself, "Oh, my arms are too flabby, oh, my thighs are too fat, oh, my skin is getting wrinkles, oh, my hair is gray," and on and on. This is not a good way to start your day! This mental abuse will leave you hopeless. When you feel like bingeing, you'll binge. What does it matter anyway? This terribly destructive pattern can be stopped if you'll slowly start to focus on your positives. Perhaps people have said you have beautiful eyes. Don't respond with your usual sarcasm. Say thanks, and absorb the good feeling. Try to slowly shift your focus in the mirror every morning from negatives to positives. Flabby arms and large hips will very slowly give way to beautiful eyes and skin. Of course your weight problem will still be there. The big difference, however, will be it won't rule your life and cause you to be depressed all the time. Experiment with the following ideas to make this transition from a negative self-focus to a positive self-image permanent:

776. *Eliminate criticism centers.* In other words, stop associating with people who criticize you, such as a hypercritical friend.

777. *Focus on making yourself the most accomplished person you can be.* Let your life revolve around becoming a better guitarist, photographer, writer, or worker each day, rather than on your appearance. This will do wonders for your self-respect and self-image.

778. *List your best qualities.* Write out a list of your best talents and qualities. It's better to focus on improving good qualities than on eliminating weak ones.

779. *Consider joining a support group.* You may benefit from working together with other people who are also trying to enhance their self-esteem.

780. *Don't let others take advantage of you.* Your self-image lowers every time you feel as if someone is taking advantage of you. This can lead to anger and resentment. To avoid this, work on saying no when you mean no and yes when you mean yes. Don't get angry and frustrated at other people. Just practice making only those commitments that you freely choose to make.

781. **Self-talk your way to a great attitude.** "Attitude is everything." But how do you improve something as intangible as attitude? One solution that works is called *self-talk*. Self-talk involves saying simple positive phrases to yourself over and over. Here are some phrases to start you out:

782. *"I'm doing the best I can."*

783. *"I can do anything I set my mind to."*

784. *"Relax."*

785. *"There are lots of things I can eat."*

786. *"I'm proud of myself."*

787. *"I like myself."*

788. **Avoid imperatives, and just do your best.** Avoid words such as *never, always,* or *must* in your internal thinking. Using these words

can lead to periods of depression and bingeing. Don't be so rigid that you can't allow yourself to slip up a little now and then. Banish phrases such as, "I will *never* eat another piece of chocolate again," or "I will *always* exercise every morning," or "I *must* always control my eating." Two strategies that will help you become more flexible are relaxed breathing and self-talk. Whenever you feel you did something you shouldn't have, take two or three deep slow breaths and then repeat to yourself a phrase such as, "Everything's going to be all right; relax; you're going to succeed," or "I'm doing the best I can. I'll try to do better next time." If you do this long enough it will become second nature, and you'll be more likely to respond to problems with relaxed breathing and relaxed thinking, instead of getting angry with yourself for not being superhuman.

789. **Adopt an attitude of prevention.** Avoid saying to yourself, "I really need this; I'm going to eat it. I'll lose it later." It's a hundred times easier to maintain your weight than it is to gain weight and then try to lose it permanently later! Always focus on prevention. Don't fool yourself into thinking you'll lose it later when things are better. There are probably always going to be complications in your life that make overeating tempting. No matter how much you're overweight, or how bleak life appears, always focus on prevention. Instead of saying, "I'll lose it later," try saying, "I don't want it now."

790. **Remember that nothing tastes as good as being trim and fit feels.** Being trim and fit feels fantastic. You have more energy and confidence, walk a bit taller, and feel generally wonderful about being the best person possible. Visualize this feeling and keep it in your head when you think you may want to stuff a high-fat treat into your mouth.

791. **Make your weight loss tangible.** Find items you can stack someplace in your home that will physically represent your extra weight. These could be weights, magazines, books, or one-pound bags of rice or beans. Whenever you lose a pound, remove its

weight equivalent from your Fat Stack and put it into a Fat-Loss Stack nearby. Watching your weight move from the Fat Stack to the Fat-Loss Stack can be very motivating.

792. **Try not to focus on only weight loss for motivation.** Too often people focus on just the idea of losing weight, and forget all of the other positive things that happen to them as by-products of their successful weight control. My study of more than 1,000 weight-control success stories revealed that, in many instances, after the person lost weight he or she then went on to succeed in other areas of life. It was common for these people to return to school, become successful at a hobby or interest, or change their careers for the better. Some even became professional fitness instructors! Why does this happen? It happens because the skills you learn losing weight are universal skills you can apply to many areas of your life. To commit to a long-term goal, plan how you're going to reach that goal, and set smaller goals that lead up to larger goals and ultimately to the final goal is to do what it takes to succeed at anything in life. So, if you're contemplating losing weight for your health, for your appearance, or just for your general happiness, don't forget that in the process you're also going to grow as a person and emerge not only healthier, but also a true achiever.

793. **Make yourself more beautiful now.** Don't wait to make yourself more beautiful until you've lost your weight. Make yourself beautiful so that you *can* lose your weight. Low self-esteem is one of the biggest problems with weight control. One way to boost your self-esteem is to make yourself more beautiful when you start your weight-control program. It might take a little money to get the look you deserve, but the results will rapidly raise your self-esteem and self-respect.

794. **Dress yourself thin.** Dressing thin may give you the visual boost you need to overcome a critical plateau and go on to achieve weight-control success. You can use a number of techniques that

revolve around colors, designs, textures, and lines to look as slender as possible. Experiment with the following ideas:

795. *Use slenderizing colors.* There are three different dimensions of color to keep in mind. The first is called *value*. Value is best described by words such as lightness and darkness. Ask yourself, what is the lightness or darkness of the color you're considering? For slenderizing, darker shades of color work best. The second dimension of color is called *hue* and is the true name that a color receives. The best hues for slenderizing are cool colors such as purple, blue, or green. The third dimension of color is called *intensity*. Intensity covers the spectrum from dull to bright. The brighter the intensity, the larger you'll appear.

796. *Use flattering lines.* Lines work well because they create optical illusions that project a feeling of height rather than width. Long and narrow pointed collars, long and narrow V necklines, diagonal lines, and vertical lines have a slimming effect.

797. *Use small patterns.* Choose patterns with small and closely spaced designs. Large patterns over a lot of space will make you look larger.

798. *Choose smooth textures.* A smooth-textured fabric will hide irregularities. For example, try shantung, linen, flannel, crepe, wool challis, or lightweight tweed.

799. *Emphasize your chest or bust to make your waist appear smaller.* Tops with patterns, cuts, or accents such as ruffles that lead the eye to your chest tend to minimize your waistline.

800. **Wear attractive clothing to stay slim.** Once you've lost your weight you may find it helpful to wear clothing you look great in, and in the summer spend time in shorts and half-cut T-shirts. The admiring looks you get may give you the confidence and motivation you need to keep the weight off.

Overcoming Difficulties

801. Reconsider whether you should be staying home all day. Many people are very active before they start to have children. They take long bike rides and walk with their mates in the evening, stay out late dancing, and wake up early to get the most out of the new day. Then the children arrive. By the time the second child turns four years old, mom or dad may barely manage to take care of the kids and fix the meals, let alone clean the house as well. If any of this sounds familiar, you may want to consider whether you should be staying home all day long. Just as an experiment, try giving yourself some breathing space during the day or at least a couple of times a week. You could trade baby-sitting with friends, have your spouse or a relative baby-sit for a few hours, try a preschool or morning day care, or have a morning or evening out. Perhaps by giving yourself some time away from the home and children the quality of your time with the kids will improve, not to mention the quality of your own life.

802. Curb depression with a happy room. Do you feel depressed and consider bingeing when it's cold and gloomy? Try turning one room in your house into a "happy room." Paint it with bright colors, hang plants all over, buy lots of big bright lights, and generally try to give the room a comfortable feel. Place past achievements on the walls and anything else that produces happy feelings in you. Next time you start to get depressed, go to your happy room—it may lift your mood.

803. Get out of the house and beat the blah blahs. The blah blahs are best defined by the word *sluggish*. You land on the couch in front of the TV with a pint of ice cream and wonder if you're ever going to get up. Needless to say, you want to try to avoid the blah blahs because they can cause bingeing. What's a solution? Get out of the house! The key? Advance planning. Realize that if you've experienced the blah blahs in the past, you're probably going to experience them again, and be prepared. First, communicate your feelings to your family. Let them know it's vital you leave the house as soon as the blah blahs hit. Tell them that it's not their fault, that sometimes for reasons you can't explain you just get the blah blahs. After you've cleared your escape with your family, plan places you can go once you leave the house. You could go over to a friend's house for support, to a place for a special walk, to the mall, the library, or a bookstore. If you have young children, you also need to find a baby-sitter who can come over at a moment's notice, or a baby-sitter where you can drop off your kids on short notice. Once you've done the planning, pay attention to your energy level. If you reach the point where you feel as if you can hardly get off the couch, and you're thinking about raiding the fridge, then don't hesitate to get out of the house. Go to your preplanned destinations and spend as much time there as you need. When the worst of the blah blahs has passed, congratulate yourself. You can feel good about having prevented a major binge. It's helpful also to spend the day after with friends or out shopping, walking, or whatever. This will improve your energy level and build on what you did the day before.

804. **Beat the morning blah blahs.** The morning blah blahs are a specific variation of the general blah blahs just described. Experiment with the strategies listed in Tips 805 through 813 to prevent them:

805. *Eat breakfast out.* Just the thought of no breakfast dishes may give you enough of a boost to get you up and out the door.

806. *Place your phone by the bed and call a friend.* Have a chat, talk about your blah blahs, and arrange to meet for breakfast or lunch.

807. *Have your shoes and walking or running stuff handy.* If you awake with the morning blah blahs, you can put them on and get out of the house and into the morning air for a quick workout as soon as possible.

808. *Plan to do something different and special with your hair.*

809. *Plan something new and different with your nails and makeup.*

810. *Run out of the house with your goal being to reach a plant or flower shop.* Plants and flowers are wonderful for a mental boost.

811. *Compose a neat and concise list of what you want to accomplish during the day.* Once you have the list in front of you, you'll feel more confident and energetic about accomplishing your goals that day.

812. *Put on a pot of decaf tea or coffee, curl up with your mate or favorite pet, and read a book.*

813. *Dress in a wacky outfit, make funny faces, or set an ambush for someone in your house.* Be creative and think of fun things you can do to spice up your morning with laughter.

814. Cope with PMS. It probably comes as no surprise that just before menstruation is when many women are most vulnerable to bingeing. Tips 815 through 819 will help you reduce your premenstrual symptoms:

815. *Limit your sugar, salt, caffeine, and alcohol intake.* Yes, that means you need to limit your chocolate escapes. Chocolate is a concentrated source of both caffeine and sugar, which can increase your moodiness and make you susceptible to bingeing. Caffeine is also a no-no if you're tired a lot. Caffeine reduces B-complex vitamins and therefore actually reduces your energy level over several hours. It can also accentuate your moodiness. As you probably already know, too much salt will cause you to retain water, bloat, and feel generally fat and disgusting. Alcohol should also be limited, since your body may not tolerate it as well during PMS.

816. *Eat a lot of little meals.* Eat four to six small and nutritionally balanced meals each day to give yourself a more consistent blood-sugar level. To stabilize your mood swings, you have to stabilize your blood sugar. Avoid going for more than three hours without a small meal or snack during PMS.

817. *Eat more B-complex-rich foods.* Eat whole-grain pastas and breads to get plenty of B-complex vitamins and you'll feel more alert and stable. Not only will you receive energy from these foods, but complex carbohydrates also help to stabilize blood-sugar levels. Green leafy veggies, liver, and legumes are also excellent sources of B vitamins.

818. *Drink eight glasses of water daily.* You should always do this, but it's particularly important during PMS. Water will flush excess salt from your body so that you don't feel bloated.

819. *Walk.* Moderate exercise keeps blood-sugar levels stable. A *minimum* workout of 15 to 20 minutes every other day during PMS might work well.

820. **Learn to cope with setbacks.** Let's face it, life is tough and setbacks are going to happen. Of course, your future always looks rosy when you first start your weight-control program. You'll have your goals all set and be ready to go and optimistic. Then life will throw you a curve such as the flu, a winter storm, or a hurt child, or your spouse will experience a crisis, and the next thing you know it will be all you can do to get through the day! Two strategies that work well here are planning and self-talk:

821. *Planning for setbacks.* A little advance mental preparation before you start will help you cope with life's inevitable setbacks. Make a list of common problems and setbacks that you think might occur, and then try to figure out in advance what you'll do when they happen. For instance, sometimes your spouse has to work late. When this happens you miss your dance class. What you can do is find three baby-sitters who say they're usually available during your dance time and will sit for you with very short notice. Obviously you aren't going to be able to plan for every setback, but doing just a little planning should help.

822. *Practice positive self-talk.* When you experience a setback that's beyond your control, try saying to yourself, "Setbacks happen;

I'll just do the best I can" or, "I'm doing the best that I can." You can't control everything in your life, no matter how hard you try. But you can always try to be your very best. As a frail human buffeted about on the often stormy sea of life, if you're sincerely struggling to do your best, then you should be proud and at ease with yourself.

823. **Ignore grim statistics.** The often-cited statistic that 90 percent of people who try to lose weight fail to do so permanently is not accurate. This statistic is based on research done in a hospital clinic more than 30 years ago! Hospital weight-loss programs attract the people who are most likely to regain their weight, and are therefore not representative of the average population. The truth is, at the moment no one knows how well average people perform when they try to lose weight. Leading experts such as Yale Professor of Psychology Kelly Brownell, Ph.D., do believe, however, that most people control their weight better than statistics show. For now the best thing to do is ignore grim statistics, try your very best, and see what happens.

824. **Realize genes don't make weight control futile.** Yes, everyone does have a biological set point. This set point is a kind of center point around which your weight fluctuates, and genetics do make it easier for some people to turn down their set points than others. But obesity is not a trait like eye color, which you're born with and doesn't ever change. You inherit a *tendency* for obesity. Genes are only one of three primary factors that make people overweight. The other two are diet and your level of physical activity. Research has proven that you definitely can lower your body's set point through exercise and diet. A recent study by the National Institutes of Health clearly showed how diet and physical activity could overcome genes. In this study, the body weights of the Pima Indians living in Arizona were compared with the body weights of their genetic counterparts in Maycoba, Mexico. The female Maycoba Pimas, despite the same genes as the Arizona Pimas, weighed 40 pounds less than the Arizona Pimas. The Maycoba men

weighed 65 pounds less than the Arizona Pimas! The difference? The Maycoba Pimas ate a diet high in complex carbohydrates, with only 20 percent of calories from fat. This represented half the fat intake of the Arizona Pimas. The Maycoba Pimas were also much more active during the day, doing lots of walking and manual work. You can't trade your body for a new one, but you can strive to be your personal best through diet and exercise. Gradually make your body as lean and muscular as possible through changes in diet and exercise, and you'll do much to enhance your appearance and quality of life.

825. **Try not to compare yourself with a social ideal.** With the constant flood of images of perfect people in mass media, it's easy to become depressed and lose confidence in your ability to look like *that*. Constantly comparing yourself with these "perfect people" will slowly erode your probably already low confidence level until you finally give up. Try to end this destructive behavior by losing weight not only for appearance, but also to improve your health and quality of life. If you are a woman, keep in mind that surveys show men prefer women with bigger hips than women think they do, and men also prefer women with smaller breasts than women think they do. In other words, women think they should have bigger breasts and smaller hips than men do! The opposite is also true. Men think most women prefer huge shoulders and massive muscles, when actually most women prefer athletic men who are moderately muscled.

826. **Reduce housework-related depression.** *Depressing. Boring. Demeaning.* These words probably come to mind when you think of housework. Surely you didn't plan on growing up and getting married only to become the cook and cleaning person for your family. Even with a career, this role might make you so depressed that you binge often as an escape. Here are some tips that should help:

827. *Focus on prevention.* The best way to reduce housework is to focus on preventing it in the first place, not on trying to do it better. Consequently the tips that follow aim to lessen housework.

828. *Put industrial entrance mats at every door in your home.* Don't skimp on these. Buy the sturdy nylon fiber mats you see at the entrances to supermarkets, offices, and other commercial buildings. Why nylon? Because using nylon in mats is like running a vacuum cleaner over everyone's shoes as they enter your doorway. Nylon creates a static charge that actually helps pull particles from your shoes.

829. *Keep your decorations few and simple.* A good tactic here is to rotate your decorations. Start by taking most of your decorations down and putting them in storage. Keep out a few pieces you really appreciate, and then focus on enjoying them. When you grow tired of them after a month or so, replace them with the other items you previously placed in storage. You'll enjoy your decor more and have less decor to clean.

830. *Do what it takes to organize your bathroom.* Buy extra towel racks to keep wet towels off the floor. Buy toothbrush holders, comb organizers, and shaving containers. Install all the extra shelf space you need so that people can find what they need without wrecking what you just finished organizing. Use liquid soap containers and get rid of the soap "stew" by your sinks. If you don't have enough drawer space, use baskets or a big crock to store grooming things. Once all the junk in your bathroom is out of the way, you'll be amazed at how quickly you can clean it.

831. *Create an organization center in each room.* In every room have a little shelf, out of reach of children, on which you can place all of your important things such as keys, the checkbook, "to do" lists, and so forth.

832. *Open up your kitchen.* Don't be afraid to hang your most-used utensils from the ceiling and on walls. Have you ever seen a pro-

fessional cook's kitchen at a gourmet restaurant? You can be sure they don't have their cooking equipment in the back of some cupboard. Have your cooking items out in the open where you can find and use them.

833. *Get appropriate kitchen storage containers.* There are more different kinds of storage containers today than ever before. They're strong, inexpensive, and lightweight. If you need to store items, go buy some. They stack well, cost little, and last forever.

834. *Buy a Don Aslett book.* There are hundreds of other things you can do to reduce your housework that are beyond the scope of this book. Do yourself a favor and buy Don Aslett's *500 Terrific Ideas for Cleaning Everything.*

835. *Don't be bullied by advertisers.* Did you know that despite countless labor-saving innovations over the past century, homemakers today spend more time cleaning than they did one hundred years ago! Vacuum cleaners, deodorizers, disinfectants, new dish soaps and clothing detergents, electric washing machines and clothes dryers, new scrub brushes, dishwashers, and so forth haven't reduced the total time people spend cleaning house. Why? Largely because over the decades advertisers for these products have annually launched campaigns to make you think you need to keep your home cleaner and cleaner. In her fascinating book *More Work for Mother: The Ironies of Household Technology from the Open Hearth to the Microwave,* historian Ruth Shwartz Cowan shows that advertisers play on the guilt of homemakers to get them to buy new products and services! Advertisers want you to think, "If my home isn't spotless, I'm a bad mother or father." Don't let them make you feel guilty or embarrassed. Keep your home functional, but try not to go to extremes. Life is too short to waste it keeping your home immaculate. Instead, spend time with your lover, friends, or children, exercising, or on self-improvement. The result will be a much more relaxed and happy person. If an overly critical friend

or relative says your house is a wreck, let him or her read your copy of *More Work for Mother*.

836. **Reduce clutter.** If you pay attention to the housework you do, you'll be surprised how much of it is caused by junk. Housework experts estimate that as much as 50 percent of your housework is caused by clutter. Eliminate your clutter and you could cut your housework by 50 percent! Try the following:

    837. *Eliminate clutter collectors such as unneeded tables.* Cut back on your table space, and the clutter will follow.

    838. *Start small.* Take it one drawer and closet at a time or you'll be overwhelmed.

    839. *Don't get sidetracked.* Concentrate on what you're doing, finish it, and then move on to something else.

    840. *Get junk out of the house the same day.* If you don't, you may reconsider the next day.

    841. *Shrink mementos.* Tired of dusting old trophies? Take a picture of you with them and then trash or store them. Save a Boy Scout badge, not the entire uniform. Blow up pictures of you in the old high-school letter jacket and then throw or give it away.

    842. *Dump it all out.* Dump the contents of the shelf, drawer, or box out onto the floor. This will force you to consider everything.

    843. *Before birthdays or holidays, clear out older toys and give them to charity.*

    844. *Two for one.* Every time you by a new pair of shoes, toy, tape cassette or CD, or garment get rid of two older ones.

845. **Use a "fat bank" to cope with high-calorie snack environments.** Next time you're standing in line at the grocery store and feel like munching on a high-calorie snack, take the money and delegate it to a "fat bank" you have at home instead. Your fat bank could be a glass jar, or an old-fashioned piggy bank. Place the money in

your fat bank and watch it grow each week. It will make your efforts tangible and save you money at the same time!

846. **Carry a goal card for a constant reminder.** Take a minute to write your goals on the back of a business card. For example, you could start by writing neatly on the back of a card:

Self-confidence
Clothes
Health
Control
Energy

Now place this card, or numerous cards, in your wallet, checkbook, or glove box, on a nightstand, or anywhere else you think appropriate. This will make your goals both tangible and visually accessible. If necessary, rewrite your card with different goals as your weight control progresses.

12.

Tips on Dealing with Friends

847. Be prepared with strategies to cope with holidays, parties, and special events. If you often overeat during holiday gatherings, parties, and special events, then experiment with the strategies in Tips 848 through 853:

848. *Tell white lies to food-pushers.* Next time someone pushes food on you, respond with, "That looks fantastic. Unfortunately for me my stomach has been upset all day and I just don't think I'd better eat any right now, but thanks for making it. It really does look wonderful." Of course, you don't need to do this with close friends. A close friend should know about your weight-control program, and together you should be helping each other by preparing light meals whenever you get together.

849. *Time your eating so that you finish your meal just after everyone else.*

850. *Serve yourself last.* At a buffet, stand around and chat while munching on veggie sticks until everyone else has been served, and then serve yourself. At a table, don't start eating until everyone has been served.

851. *Call ahead to find out what you'll be eating.* You can use this information to create a tentative list of what you expect to eat, and then add up the calories and fat grams to see how they fit into your daily calorie and fat-gram goals.

852. *Focus on unique tastes.* Focus your eating on unique tastes that you don't experience at home.

853. *Use all of your senses, eat slowly, and enjoy every single bite.*

854. **Write a friend to beat depression.** Why not write a long letter to one of your close friends to pinpoint the cause of your depression? This keeps you in contact with your friends and helps your depression because, through writing your thoughts down, you can clearly identify the cause of your depression and so deal with it more effectively. Also, by your sitting down and dealing with your problems immediately they don't get out of control.

855. **Make peer pressure work for you.** It happens. You finally start to lose weight and your overweight friends feel threatened and start to pressure you in myriad ways to stay fat like them. If you find yourself in this situation, remember that your friends are doing this because they're frightened. They're scared to death you're going to lose all your excess weight and live happily ever after and leave them fat, alone, and miserable. Try not to explode at them and jeopardize your relationship. Take time to talk with them to let them know how you feel. If your attempts at communication don't work, take all of the negative energy and anger your friends are generating in you and focus it into a weight-control positive such as dancing or lifting weights. By venting your frustration through fitness, you'll burn calories, reduce stress, and be less likely to explode angrily at your friends.

856. **Fix for your guests what you'd fix for yourself.** Don't go berserk and fix all sorts of high-fat foods when you have guests over to eat. You'll gain five pounds cleaning up afterwards. If you feel you must do some high-fat baking, then send all the leftovers home with your guests, freeze some, give them to a neighbor, or discard them.

857. **Request healthy food when someone else buys.** You don't have to eat every high-fat dish in the restaurant just because someone else is paying for it. Go ahead and treat yourself to some expensive tastes—just don't overdo it. As a little added insurance, ask to go to a healthy restaurant.

858. **Tell others about your weight-control efforts.** Weight control is so difficult that it only makes sense that you should enlist the support and help of as many people as you can. If you really want to lose your weight and keep it off, be willing to risk failing in front of other people. Talking to others will positively affect your weight control in a number of ways. It will not only have the effect of creating a network of support, but it will also make your goal much more concrete. Talking constantly about your goal to everyone will transform it from a dream into an everyday reality, and others will respect you for your efforts.

859. **Avoid eating something just because your friend is.** You don't have to eat the same thing your friend is to make your friend comfortable. Just because she has decided to eat a hot fudge sundae, that doesn't mean you have to order one too. A true friend will feel comfortable with whatever you're eating.

860. **Burn fat while you socialize.** Do you get together with your friends three or so times a week to chat, eat, and socialize? Why not combine your socializing with working out? Instead of getting together to eat and complain about your weight, start getting together to walk, cycle, or dance. This way you'll get the best of both worlds. You'll receive support from one another to work out consistently, and you'll socialize, too.

861. **Change the friends you play with.** Have you noticed that your children's behavior is dictated in large part by the kinds of friends they play with? If they spend time with smokers, it's almost inevitable they'll try cigarettes. It's no different with adults. Consequently when starting your weight-control program, develop a network of health-conscious friends by participating in clubs that

revolve around healthy activities. For instance, if you like hiking, there are hiking clubs all over the country you can join. The same is true for walking, dancing, skiing, biking, and so forth. Take some time to track these people down. Once you find them you'll have access to a large support network of people bonded together by their love for a particular activity. Soon you'll be going to events together, eating together, and feeding off each other's energy. This will do wonders for your mind and body.

862. **Use a people fix to avoid depression.** Watching people in itself can be entertaining and comforting. Next time you're depressed and alone, try heading straight for the nearest public place for a people fix. It could be a grocery store, a park, a farmer's market, or perhaps a shopping mall. It doesn't matter. Just get out and among some other humans for a while, and use the time to identify the cause of your depression.

863. **Prioritize your relationships to avoid people traps.** Some people can never say no to the demands of friends and acquaintances. This pattern of always trying to please others and of taking on too much responsibility will ultimately burn you out. One thing you can do that should help is to prioritize your relationships. Write out a list of the people in your life. Carefully think about your relationships with them, and then list them in their order of importance to you. Next, do the same thing for the various groups to which you belong. Start your recovery by dealing only with people and groups at the top of your lists. When you speak with the people low on your lists, politely say no over and over to them until you've freed yourself of all but your most important obligations. Right away you'll have more time for personal fitness, to spend with your family, and for the people and groups that matter most in your life.

864. **Try not to withdraw from the world.** Realize that by withdrawing into your own private world of depression you're only making your loneliness and depression worse. You have to take action

to make friends. You can't presume good friends will just appear. You need to find situations where you can meet people who share a mutual interest. To meet people you'll want to reach out to, join a club that centers on an activity. This is an almost guaranteed formula for meeting and developing new friends. After you've met someone you like, invite him or her to join you at a concert, sporting event, or other pastime that doesn't focus on food.

13.

Tips on Taking Charge of Your Weight Loss

Before You Begin

865. Make certain you're ready with a pro/con list and two-week trial. Motivation in people tends to ebb and flow over time. You may actually be preventing a failure by choosing to lose weight later. It's best to start your weight-control effort during a period of peak motivation. A pro/con list for losing weight is a good way to do this. In one column, place the benefits you'll derive from losing weight. In another column, place the negative things that could occur if you tried to lose weight. Benefits could include things such as more energy, a better social life, a wider variety of clothing, self-confidence, improved health, or a better chance for a job or a date. In your negative column be completely honest with yourself and write down *all* of the negatives. List things such as irritability, threatened friends and family, perceived hunger, and problems with eating out, at social situations, during the holidays, and so forth. After you have this pro/con list, carefully think about whether or not you're sufficiently motivated at this time to tackle the negatives. Do the positives motivate you enough that you'll be able to overcome the negatives? If not, then wait a few weeks, write up another pro/con list, and see how you feel at that time. While waiting, comfort yourself with the knowledge that you may be preventing a future failure. If, after writing a pro/con list, you're still unsure whether or not you're really motivated, take a two-week trial of exercising more and consuming fewer calories and fat grams. Say to yourself, "Okay, I'll try it for just two weeks to see how it goes." The success you experience during this trial period may be enough to motivate you to continue with your efforts.

866. **Don't start by adding up all the diets you've been on in the past.** This is a very depressing and destructive way to start a weight-control program.

867. **Buy this book.** If you're reading a friend's copy of this book and enjoy what you're reading, then take a minute to buy a copy for yourself. This is a quick-reference guidebook packed with an enormous amount of information that you just can't use effectively when you borrow it briefly. The book costs about as much as a large pizza, but in sharp contrast to a large pizza it will effectively help you lead a healthier and happier life through better weight control for years to come.

868. **Cope with emotional sabotage from the start.** Whether it's losing weight or contemplating a career change, any major lifestyle decision you try to make is vulnerable to emotional sabotage. Tips 869 through 873 will help you cope with emotional sabotage so that you don't doom your weight-loss effort with a wishy-washy commitment:

869. *Guilt.* Guilt that stems from a perceived failure to fulfill familial duties as a direct result of weight-loss activity often prevents people from committing to weight loss. For example, Mark picks the kids up after school and would feel guilty if his wife took on that responsibility so that he could go for a walk. Barbara does all the cooking and grocery shopping and would feel guilty if her husband had to cook and shop so that she could swim. A good strategy here is to sit down together with your spouse and list all of your responsibilities to see exactly who is doing what on the home

front. Gallup research shows typically women do the laundry 88 percent of the time, cook 85 percent of the time, do the dishes 83 percent of the time, make the beds 82 percent of the time, grocery shop 81 percent of the time, vacuum 80 percent of the time, and pay bills 58 percent of the time. Typically men will wash the car and mow the grass. If you are a woman in a typical household, then you shouldn't feel the least bit guilty about asking your husband to do more around the house so that you can devote more time to weight control. Try dividing jobs so that both of you do the jobs you like. Also try rotating jobs neither of you like monthly. When one of you starts a new job, be sure the other doesn't nag or criticize. Be patient with your partner, and keep in mind that proficiency at a new task takes time.

870. *Worry.* At first Mary thought she really needed to lose weight and was ready to make a commitment to weight loss. But then, the more she thought about it, the more she began to worry about every little thing. She worried she would spend too much money on equipment and clothing. She worried she couldn't afford to buy new clothing when she lost weight. She even worried that her husband would become jealous of other men eyeing her once she lost weight! If you do nothing long enough, it's easy to create so many perceived problems that you decide to forget the whole thing. Make your decision and act on it. Otherwise, you may never take action. Deal with problems as they arise—if they ever do.

871. *Perfectionism.* If you're a perfectionist, you may have trouble deciding whether or not to lose weight because you don't have a color-coordinated running suit for when it rains. Maybe you think the 20 or 30 articles and dozen or so books you've read on weight loss aren't enough to get you started, and you want to read just a few more. Maybe you think you're not fast enough to run in public, trendy enough to go to aerobics, or coordinated enough to show your face in dance class. Try not to think about these things. Successful weight control is an attitude. What really counts is that

you have a determined and positive mental outlook. Also, remember that most people have tremendous respect for a person trying to learn something new. They realize that no one is perfect from the start. So don't worry if you happen to look a little foolish when you first learn a new weight-control activity. Have fun. If anyone does happen to make a negative comment, remember, that person's the one with the problem, not you.

872. *Procrastination.* Human beings have a remarkable capacity for rationalizing procrastination. An annual rationalization pattern for putting off weight loss might proceed as follows:

January—"I'll wait until spring to lose weight when the weather is nicer and I've recovered from the holidays."
April—"I'm really busy getting ready for summer, and besides, when the summer comes the days will be longer and I'll have more time to exercise."
August—"Summer's over, so I no longer need to look good in skimpy clothing. I also have to get the kids ready for school, and we're going on a vacation this month, so I'll wait until fall."
November—"I'm really busy preparing for the holidays and all the relatives, and I can never control my eating over the holidays anyway, so I'm going to wait until after the new year."

The next thing you know another year has come and gone and you still haven't sincerely tried to lose weight. Realize that if you don't want to commit to weight control, it's very easy to come up with a thousand excuses. Also realize, however, that if you *do* want to commit to weight control, starting can be as easy as putting on your sneakers and going for a casual walk tonight.

873. *Fear.* While many emotions can sabotage your decision to lose weight, fear is the emotion that's usually most problematic. Fear of failure is part of the emotional anxiety surrounding any major decision, and the decision to lose weight is no exception. When

confronting this emotion, it's helpful to keep in mind that failure is a part of the human experience. Try not to view failure as a negative, but rather as an opportunity to learn and improve yourself so that you can do better next time. Almost no one is instantly successful at anything in life. Rather, success is the product of experience gained through constant trial and error. Why should your success story be any different? Expect to experience setbacks. But also expect that if you keep learning from your mistakes, it's almost inevitable that at some point you'll succeed.

874. **Write out a contract.** Contracts work well for many people. They make your goals more tangible and real. You can make focused contracts for ideas such as learning three new recipes a week, or you can make more general contracts for categories such as fitness, food, or behavior. Do whatever makes you feel most comfortable. For example, if you wrote a fitness contract, over the next month you could plan to swim three times a week for 20 minutes at a time. Write this goal down and write down when and where you're going to swim. Next, sign and date your contract and make photocopies for friends and family. To finish, figure out how you'll reward yourself for your success. A good place to start is with the nonfood rewards listed in Tips 946 through 957.

875. **Find more time for weight control.** You may be a wife, mother of two, businessperson, cook, house cleaner, designated errand runner, payer of bills, and many other things to other people. Of course your weight problem is going to stem in large part from a simple lack of time. Experiment with the ideas in Tips 876 through 889 to find more time for weight control:

876. *Wake up 20 minutes earlier and go to bed 20 minutes later.* Try it for a week to see if you miss the extra 40 minutes of sleep. You probably won't, and in the process you'll have created another 40 minutes of time for yourself during the day. Specifically, try getting out of bed shortly after you open your eyes. As soon as you

open your eyes, focus on the very best thing that's going to happen to you that day, and use this thought to get out of bed.

877. *Shower.* A shower uses one-third less time than a bath.

878. *Use meal trays.* Place cups, silverware, and plates on trays that can be taken by family members to the table in one trip.

879. *Make priority lists.* Try making a list of everything you want to accomplish the next day each evening before you go to sleep. List your activities from most to least important. If you don't accomplish something that's been at the bottom of your list for several days, often you can just scratch it off as unimportant.

880. *Reduce junk mail.* Read mail daily by a recycling bin, and have your name removed from mailing lists by writing the Direct Marketing Association, P.O. Box 9008, Farmingdale, NY 11735, and asking to have your name removed by the mail-preference service.

881. *Use detailed organization and planning.* Make a list of long-term goals (five years) that you want to achieve. Next, break down each of these goals into smaller goals that can be achieved at three years and at one year, then into still smaller goals that can be achieved quarterly, then monthly, and finally weekly. Using detailed planning you'll make good use of your time during the day, week, month, and year so that you'll have more time for fitness.

882. *Question repetition.* Always question repetitive acts to discover better ways to accomplish them.

883. *Reduce procrastination.* Three steps work particularly well to reduce procrastination. First, schedule your most unpleasant tasks first so that you get them out of the way. Second, commit to the deadlines you've set. Third, reward yourself after you've accomplished your goals with a nice internal phrase such as, "Nicely done."

884. *Delegate.* Avoid doing everything yourself. Think about the tasks you perform at work and at home, and figure out if you can del-

egate any of them to family or coworkers. Be sure to praise and reward those who help you.

885. **Read a book on time-saving.** If you haven't already, read *How to Gain an Extra Hour Every Day* by Ray Josephs.

886. **Watch less television.** Most of us spend about 40 percent of our leisure time watching television. That translates into between 15 and 18 hours of television a week. This is an understandable habit, since watching television is easy and *appears* relaxing. The fact is, however, research at Rutgers University suggests people actually feel less relaxed and satisfied after watching television than they did before watching it! This happens for a variety of reasons, which range from poor programs, to feeling as if you're wasting your life, to feeling guilty because you could have been productive and talked with friends, exercised, learned the guitar, read, volunteered your time for a good cause, or had a full night's sleep. Try Tips 887 to 889 to cut your time in front of the television:

   887. *Tape shows on your* VCR. This way you can skip the ads and the slow parts of the program.

   888. *Don't watch TV—watch TV shows.* Avoid mindlessly turning on the television. Use a television guide to select the shows you really want to watch and then watch only them.

   889. *Try a TV rationing machine.* One such machine is called TimeSlot. When you sign up you receive a TV "credit card" that gives you a set amount of TV time each week. You can acquire one through North Carolina Public Television at (800) 693-3939 for around $120. Another less costly device is called *TVLockOut*, and is installed between the television and the antenna. It's a lockbox that blocks all television reception with the turn of a key. It's available for around $25 from some electronics stores or by calling (800) 223-6009.

890. **Take full responsibility.** Family, friends, and true professionals often can help you lose weight, but you can't hold them or their program responsible for *your* weight. By deferring your authority

to others, you keep yourself in a passive and helpless role, unable to do what it takes to lose weight and keep it off. The reason this is so appealing, however, is that when you do this you don't have to take any responsibility, and so if you fail it's the diet's fault and you're simply a victim. How can you ever hope to solve a problem if you believe that someone else is responsible? You may get motivated to lose weight that way if you pay a lot of money or if you like someone enough, but it's unlikely you'll keep the weight off that way. You must first accept complete responsibility for your weight before you can begin to change it. The only thing victims gain in the world of weight control is weight.

891. **Forget commercial diet companies other than Weight Watchers.** The only commercial diet company I can recommend in good conscience is Weight Watchers.[9] They're relatively inexpensive, their food products and recipes are among the best, and some people find their meetings quite helpful. Hearing from people who overcame a problem similar to one you're experiencing, and just being around others who are successfully losing weight, can be very motivating. Be sure to attend several different meetings before you decide whether you want to sign up. You may find the personality of one group or leader more appealing than another. The size of the group may also affect your decision.

   If you decide to experiment with other commercial diet companies such as Jenny Craig, Diet Center, Nutri/Systems, or Diet Workshop, then use the questions in Tips 892 through 895 as part of your evaluation:

892. *Of all those who started, what percentage finished the program?*

893. *Of those who completed the program, what percentage lost weight and how much?*

---

[9]Overeaters Anonymous and TOPS (Take Off Pounds Sensibly) are not commercial diet companies. See Tip 959 for information on these organizations.

894. *How much of the lost weight did they maintain for one, three, and five years?*

895. *What percentage experienced adverse psychological or medical effects, and how severe were these effects?*

896. **When needed, seek advice from true professionals.** Many people find registered dieticians, physical fitness specialists, psychologists, and doctors to be an indispensable part of their weight control. The key here is to utilize only true professionals. For instance, beware of people in private practice, or who work for commercial diet companies, who call themselves "nutritionists." Seek diet and nutrition advice from only registered dieticians. Many commercial diet centers are staffed with nutritionists who aren't qualified to give you advice. In many states people also can call themselves "psychotherapists" without any formal training in psychology. Check the degrees and certifications of anyone with whom you wish to consult. Also, try not to be a passive participant. Read everything you can and continue to experiment with ideas you think might work for you. The more you know in general, and the more you know about yourself in particular, the better you'll be able to communicate with your health-care professional to create solutions that will work for you. Remember, you're seeking only *advice* from professionals, not absolute direction. If you don't like something, let the advisor know, and together find an alternative strategy. Otherwise you'll never stick with it. You may find the people and organizations listed in Tips 897 through 902 helpful in your search:

897. *Your personal physician.*

898. *The American Dietetic Association,* 216 W. Jackson St., Ste. 800, Chicago, IL 60606, phone (312) 899-0040; or call the Consumer Nutrition Hotline at (800) 366-1655.

899. *The American Psychological Association,* 750 First St., Washington, DC 20002; phone (800) 374-2721.

900. *International Association of Eating Disorders Professionals,* 123 N.W. 13th St., Ste. 206, Boca Raton, FL 33432; phone (407) 338-6494.

901. *The American Society of Bariatric Physicians,* 5600 S. Quebec St., Ste. 109A, Englewood, CO 80111; phone (303) 779-4833. (Bariatric physicians specialize in weight loss.)

902. *Check your local health clubs, universities, colleges, or high schools for physical fitness specialists.* These places might also give you a referral for a personal trainer, or you can call the Aerobics and Fitness Association of America at (800) 983-2677.

903. **Create a diet history so that you don't try the same thing over and over.** You may be surprised at what you discover about yourself when you write your personal diet history. Talk to family and friends, and try to make it as complete, accurate, and honest as you possibly can. Once you do this, and review your history, you may discover you've been trying the same strategies over and over again. To avoid this in the future, maintain a general weight-control history in which you keep track of all the different weight-control strategies you try.

904. **Discover how to weigh yourself.** As a general guideline, leading weight-control psychologists such as Kelly Brownell, Ph.D., recommend that you weigh yourself no less than once a week and no more than once each day. Since water retention varies from one to four pounds daily due to hormonal swings, stress, salt intake, and alcohol intake, many people who weigh themselves daily find they're on an emotional roller coaster. Others who weigh less than once a week often find it difficult to stay motivated. These, however, are merely general observations that give you a place to start. To fine-tune your weighing, experiment with different strategies and record how you feel each time after you weigh yourself. Give each weighing strategy one or two weeks. For instance, one week weigh yourself in the morning. During the next week weigh yourself in the evening. One week weigh yourself every day.

During the next week weigh yourself only once at the end of the week. Now go back over your notes to see which strategy made you happiest. For some people this means never weighing at all until, based on visual appearance, they think they've lost all their excess weight. For others this means climbing onto the scale every day. For still others this means using a measuring tape and bypassing the scale altogether. The point is you will never know, until you experiment on yourself, exactly what will work best for you as an individual. Tips 905 through 908 discuss tapes, calipers, and underwater immersion.

905. **If the scale doesn't work, try a tape measure, skin caliper, underwater immersion, or a combination.** Weight loss measured by a scale is actually an adequate indicator of fat loss for the average person. Using a scale also has the benefits of being cheap and accessible. Nevertheless some people, particularly those who often lift heavy weights, find that a scale just doesn't work well for them. They're losing fat but gaining so much muscle that their scales don't reveal their fat loss. Others have what can only be called scalephobia. Still others insist scales are primitive and outdated and shouldn't be used, even though for the average person this isn't true. Regardless of the reasons, if you don't feel comfortable using a scale, or find it doesn't work, then you shouldn't use one. Two accessible and relatively inexpensive alternatives are the tape measure and skin caliper:

906. *Tape measure.* To use a tape measure, a woman should measure her hips and right thigh weekly to monitor her progress. A man should measure his waist at similar intervals to measure his progress. Tape measures work because humans store fat in certain locations on their bodies. You can monitor your fat loss by measuring the amount of fat in these fat-storage areas. Your ultimate goal should be a healthy waist-to-hip ratio. You calculate your ratio by measuring your waist at the level of your belly button, then measuring your hips at the widest part. Divide the waist

number by the hip number. It's healthiest for women to have a ratio of 0.8 or less. Men should try to keep the ratio below 1.0.

907. *Skin calipers.* You can buy skin calipers at a fitness store as part of a home body-fat kit, measure yourself to establish a baseline, and then use them at the end of each month to see how much fat you've lost compared with your baseline. Skin calipers can be very motivating when used to monitor how much fat you're losing. Calipers won't, however, accurately measure your total body fat. They will only estimate your body fat to within 3 to 4 percent. For instance, if you produce a reading of 20, your body is 16 to 24 percent fat. To accurately measure your body fat, you'll have to use the underwater immersion method discussed next.

908. *Underwater immersion.* Although more expensive and less accessible for most people than a measuring tape or skin caliper, underwater immersion is currently the most accurate device to measure fat loss. When done correctly, it will best reflect a person's actual lean and fat content. Most midsize or larger cities will have at least one underwater immersion tank. If you're interested in using one, call local health clubs to see if you can locate one near you. If you can afford the time and money, you may want to use an underwater immersion tank once at the start of your program, and then every six months thereafter, in addition to the scale, tape, or caliper. This way you can see how much your lean body weight is increasing and your fat decreasing. Using underwater immersion testing, you should strive for the following maximum body-fat percentages:

Race	Female	Male
Caucasian	22%	15%
Black	19%	12%
Oriental	25%	18%

909. **Photograph your progress.** Instead of using a scale, measuring tape, or calipers to monitor your progress, you may find it more

effective and motivating to take pictures of yourself naked once a month.

910. **Be honest with yourself.** It's crucial that you always be completely honest with yourself during your weight-control program.

911. **Identify why you overeat.** Identifying exactly why you overeat is the first step toward effectively dealing with it. Tips 912 through 929 list common reasons people overeat. See how many of these eating behaviors apply to you. Use the list to help you consciously understand why you're overeating. Once you've made the process of overeating conscious, you can work on strategies that will help you deal with it effectively:

912. *What a deal.* All-you-can-eat shrimp with salad bar. You'd better eat them all to get your money's worth.

913. *You'll become malnourished.* If you don't eat that roast beef sandwich loaded with mayonnaise for lunch, you might become malnourished.

914. *Before and after exercise.* You're going to walk three miles bright and early in the morning, so you can go ahead and overeat tonight. Wow, you just had a really great workout. You earned that candy bar.

915. *Escape and comfort.* You've had a really hard day. You deserve that piece of cheesecake.

916. *Television eating.* One hour after you start watching TV you can't believe you ate an entire pint of ice cream. You don't even remember tasting it.

917. *Bored to death.* You're so bored you could just die, so you eat a high-fat treat to liven the day up for several minutes, knowing full well you'll be depressed about your binge 20 minutes after you're done.

918. *Guilt.* You blame yourself because your husband is failing at his job and the children are having trouble with their schooling, and so you binge.

919. *You're never satisfied.* You hate your job, your boyfriend is a jerk, and you hate the new clothes you bought. You go to the fridge again and stare at the shelves to see what you can stuff into your mouth this time for five seconds of empty and meaningless satisfaction.

920. *No one's watching.* You stuff down an ice cream bar and then hide the wrapper in the bottom of the trash can just because no one is watching.

921. *Before and after you diet.* You mistakenly believe that dieting is boring, painful, and tasteless. Consequently you binge before and after you diet.

922. *Enjoy life; live a little.* You'd better hurry and eat another banana split; you may be hit by a car getting your paper in the morning.

923. *Unique eating.* You're at a pastry shop with a friend and you discover a new dessert you've never tried before. You make a complete pig of yourself just because the dessert is new and unique.

924. *Stress.* You eat a pint of ice cream to get a handle on yourself so that you can deal with your parent-teacher conference.

925. *Special occasion.* It's a holiday, birthday, or wedding and that means you can eat all you want.

926. *It's time to eat.* It's 5:00 and that means you're hungry, even if you just ate at 4:00.

927. *Eating for later.* You think you need to eat a lot now so that you won't be hungry later. If you're preparing to participate in a full-length basketball game or triathlon, this may be true. In daily life, however, eating for later is unnecessary and often a way to rationalize overeating.

928. *You're lonely.* Perhaps your spouse has been busy working long hours, which naturally makes you lonely, but instead of finding comfort in close friends, relatives, children, or self-improvement, you try to cope with your loneliness by eating high-fat, sugary foods, which will probably make you even more depressed an hour or so after you've eaten them.

929. *Because nobody else wants it.* If nobody else wants it, you eat it. The result is it ends up as fat on your hips instead of as compost in a landfill.

930. **Identify and stop chains of events that lead to your high-risk situations.** A high-risk situation is a situation in which the chances are very good you're going to overeat. For some people it's going to mom's house for dinner. For others it's the first 30 minutes after they arrive home from work. It's helpful to first identify these kinds of situations, and then plan in advance strategies that will help you deal with them. Remember, the more frequently you give in to food cravings, the stronger they become. The best way to identify high-risk situations is to keep weight-control records, and then search them for similar situations in which you overeat again and again. Once you've used your records to identify your high-risk situations, list each one on paper. Your goal now should be to figure out each of the separate steps that led you into the situation in the first place. High-risk situations don't just happen suddenly for no reason. Rather, they're the result of a long chain of events. To illustrate this, let's examine the chain of events in the example of always overeating during the first 30 minutes after you arrive home from work:

    a. When you shopped last, you didn't have a list, and so you didn't have any healthy meals planned to eat at home.
    b. You stored cookies on your counter top.
    c. You stayed up late to watch a late-night TV show.
    d. You woke up late in the morning, and so didn't have time to eat breakfast or make a lunch.

e. As usual you were very busy during lunch, and since you didn't pack a lunch, you ended up eating fast food with a friend.

f. You arrived home devoid of nutrition and starving, and headed for the kitchen. You didn't have any healthy meals planned, and you were so hungry you headed straight for the cookie jar when you saw it and ate a dozen or so cookies.

g. Now you felt like a failure, said to yourself, "What does it matter," and ate even more cookies.

Do you see what's happening here? One event led to another, and to another, and to another, until a high-risk situation was created that, in the end, was almost unavoidable. To end this destructive chain of events, focus your efforts on planning strategies that will help you break the chain early in its development. To do this, you could list the chain of events described above in one column, and in another column next to it you could list strategies that would help you stop each event dead in its tracks. For example, your second list of chain-breaking remedies might read:

a. Start planning meals and shopping from a list.

b. Store cookies in freezer or in opaque container.

c. Go to bed on time. (Tape worthwhile shows for future viewing.) Wake up on time.

d. Fix a healthy lunch the night before, and take it to work.

e. Go to the store before you go home, buy a bagel first, eat it, then shop for a healthy dinner.

f. Practice relaxed breathing and positive self-talk so that you don't feel like such a failure when you slip up. Don't be a perfectionist.

g. Realize it's okay to make a mistake. Everyone makes mistakes. You can binge and not destroy all the hard work you've done.

Give this chain-breaking strategy a real chance. Identify, analyze, and then try to stop the chains of events that lead to your high-risk situations *as early in the process as possible.* This strategy could finally put you on the road to permanent weight control.

931. **Try not to dwell.** Don't dwell on, "How did I ever get this way?" If you don't do something, anything, you're only going to get worse, not better. Dwelling gets you nowhere.

932. **Get help from your VCR.** If you were raised on television, you may be visually oriented. Why not turn this into a weight-control positive? Your VCR could actually be your secret weapon against fat! You can use it to help with every aspect of your weight-control program, beyond just playing exercise videos. Tips 933 through 938 give some examples:

933. *Relaxation.* Put together a collection of videos you find relaxing and label them with the words "stress medicine." These could include old-favorite upbeat movies, or relaxing visual extravaganzas such as *Over New England,* a film of New England by airplane accompanied by wonderfully relaxing music. You name the vision you need to relax, and you probably can find a home video that will help you.

934. *Humor.* Few things stop a binge as well as humor. Gather tapes of stand-up comedians and funny movies to watch whenever you become depressed and feel like bingeing.

935. *Put life in perspective.* Collect tapes designed to make your everyday problems seem trivial. A classic movie for this is *It's a Wonderful Life* with Jimmy Stewart. After watching a movie like this, you'll be less likely to become upset over something in your life that's trivial.

936. *Escape.* Get tapes that let you escape and travel to distant lands. This is an excellent way to satisfy your need to escape without using food. There are many exciting and beautiful travel videos from which to choose.

937. *Activities.* Get tapes for interests such as running, mountain biking, or cross-country skiing.

938. *Self-improvement.* Acquire tapes that teach you how to low-fat cook, organize your home, fix your car, play a musical instrument, care for children, and so forth. Your public library is loaded with more instructional home videos than you'll know what to do with. Learn how to knit, dance, cycle, golf, and paint, all from your home.

939. **Use visualization to help you achieve.** Visualizing your goals in your mind is especially helpful if you're having trouble with setting and achieving goals. Here's how you do it. After you've finished your daily tasks, and you're absolutely sure you won't be distracted, find a quiet room and dim or turn off the lights. Lie down or recline in a comfortable position. Close your eyes and take deep slow breaths. Focus all your attention on your breathing. (The sound of breathing is a natural relaxant.) After you've done this for two or three minutes, start repeating to yourself the word "relax" each time you exhale with a deep slow breath. Feel your limbs and your whole body droop into a totally relaxed state. Do this "relax" breathing for about five minutes.

Now you're ready to start your visualization (don't fall asleep yet!). First visualize an empty white screen, like a large movie screen. Take your time and try to make your image of the screen as clear as you possibly can. Now place on your screen the most serene picture you can imagine. A picture with calm water in it often works well. Hold on to this calm image for about a minute, and then clear your screen back to a blank. Now you're ready to visualize your goals. You may find it effective to split up your visualization between long-term and short-term goals. A long-term goal would be a vision of you slipping your slender body into a silky new dress. A short-term goal would be a vision of you walking faster than ever, and feeling wonderful while you do it. The key here is to use all of your senses when you visualize in order to make your vision as real as possible.

See the slender and fit new you standing in front of the three-way mirror in the store dressing room.

Feel the silky smooth dress slide onto your firm new body.

Smell the store smells and the smell of your new dress.

Hear other shoppers milling about the store.

Use all of your senses and visualize your goal for about five or ten minutes, until you fall asleep, or can no longer keep a clear, powerful image in your head. It will take time, 15 minutes a day, every day for several months, but you'll know when you've succeeded. When you become proficient at visualization, your goals will be much easier to attain, because your brain is convinced you're attaining them briefly each night!

940. **Don't assume you can just exercise away whatever you eat.** Many people wrongly assume that through exercise they can burn off whatever they eat. This attitude almost inevitably leads to overeating. This becomes readily apparent when you keep a food diary. You won't believe how much high-calorie food you're eating. You may think you're eating healthy, and you may be to a large extent, but the fact will still remain that you constantly overeat. Try not to rationalize overeating because you exercise, and you'll substantially improve your weight control.

941. **Transform your obsession with food into an obsession with something else.** Are you obsessed with food? Does your entire day revolve around meals? What are you going to eat for breakfast; for lunch? What would be the perfect treat for after lunch? What should you eat for dinner? What would be the perfect dessert after dinner? You can't expect to lose weight and keep it off when you're obsessed with food. You may lose your weight, but sooner or later it's going to creep back on unless you deal with your obsession. A good solution is to become obsessed about something else! Spend time trying various interests in order to find something you love enough that you could become obsessed with it. For example, you may discover that you love gardening. You may take

a class, join a gardening club, subscribe to gardening magazines, buy gardening books, plow up a bunch of your backyard, buy terrariums, and, in short, become obsessed with gardening. Now when you wake up in the morning, you water and feed all your plants before going to work. During lunch, you read about gardening and talk about it with your gardening friends. When you come home, you rush through dinner so that you can get outside and garden before dark. After dark you work with terrariums and other things, and then do some reading before bed. Do you see what happened? With gardening, your job, your family, and your friends, you now simply have much less time for food. Once you find something other than food that you truly love and feel passionate about, that fills your imagination and dreams, your obsession with food just may gradually disappear.

While You're Doing It

942. **Vent your anger through exercise.** Many people eat compulsively because they're mad at the world. "Why me? It's not fair. Look at that skinny person over there; she can eat like a pig and not gain a pound. Who says I can't eat that? Why was I dealt this rotten hand?" they say to themselves over and over, all the while burying their anger in fatty and sugary foods. If you find yourself saying phrases such as these, then the chances are good that when you stop overeating you're going to become angry. During this time it's crucial you vent your anger and not suppress it, but at the same time you don't want to alienate your friends and family, who are easy and convenient targets for your anger. A good solution here is to vent your anger through aerobic exercise. When you feel hate welling up inside you, go for a long walk, bike ride, hike, swim, or ski, and cry or yell until you've vented your pent-up emotion through exercise. Do this as often as you need to. Your body and mind should gradually adjust to your new lifestyle, and your anger should dissipate.

943. Exercise aerobically to avoid panic attacks. A panic attack is best described as a moment when you become overwhelmed with incredibly negative, self-critical, and hopeless thoughts. Sometimes these attacks come from nowhere; other times they're the result of an ongoing depression. Whatever the cause, the result is often a binge. It's all too easy to find quick comfort and security in food during a panic situation. If you experience panic attacks, try aerobic exercise to avoid them. During aerobic exercise the body secretes endorphins, which are natural pain killers that give a person a sense of euphoria. The body also secretes certain substances that act as natural antidepressants. This combined effect is often called a "fitness high."

A fitness high is a thousand times better than a "chocolate high." After a workout such as a long, fast walk, you'll feel mentally invigorated and at the same time experience a wonderful sense of internal calm and well-being. Compare this feeling with the depression and moodiness you experience 30 minutes after you've eaten a piece of chocolate. There's a letting-go, a warmth, and a deep relaxation that you experience after aerobic exercise that helps you sleep well at night and feel stable during the day. Even better, these positive effects last about 24 hours, depending on the intensity and duration of your workout.

944. Avoid buying clothing four sizes too small. Buy slenderizing clothing as a reward for your progress through your weight loss or as an incentive to help you feel confident and motivated when you first start. Don't, however, buy something that's too small. What inevitably happens is you try it on too soon. You then become depressed because it of course doesn't fit. Instead, it graphically illustrates that you aren't losing your weight as fast as you would like. The result is depression and low self-confidence, and the next thing you know you're off your weight-control program.

945. Reward yourself without food. Most people know they shouldn't reward themselves with food, yet it's very difficult to avoid this behavior. One solution is to make a quick-reference list of non-food rewards you'll find satisfying. The ideas in Tips 946 through 957 are guidelines you can use to create your own personal list of nonfood rewards:

946. *Clothing to make losing easier.* Usually popular articles will advise you to buy an evening dress or suit when you've finally done it. But what about rewards for your first goals, say, after you lose the first 10 or 20 pounds? Here it works best to save the expensive silk dresses for later, when you've lost all your weight, and to buy exercise clothing. What better way to reward yourself than with new clothing that will make your exercise more comfortable, safe, and appealing?

947. *A fun and fit trip.* You don't have to spend thousands of dollars and fly for days to enjoy traveling. Just travel to a regional attraction for a weekend. Early in your weight-control program make every effort to combine your reward with some form of weight-control activity. For example, if you love to mountain bike, why not reward yourself with a trip to a place with a beautiful mountain bike trail? Your local bookstore or library will have guidebooks for whatever activity you pursue. Read some and plan a trip to an exciting new place that will be fun and a good workout at the same time. If you're single, go with a friend, share a room, and split the costs. If you're married with children, share babysitting with another couple so that you can go one weekend and they can go the next.

948. *Strong-scented flowers.* Buy flowers that have strong and pleasant scents to make it the most sensual experience possible. Roses are a typical favorite.

949. *The right equipment will make losing easier.* Go buy those cross-country skis you've been meaning to buy for five years for your reward. Having the equipment for your activities will help you lose weight.

950. *Not just any bubble bath.* Go to a bath specialty shop and buy some unique soaps and bubble baths to make your bath an experience in luxurious satisfaction. Lock the door and lock out the world for a while.

951. *Light recipes.* Light recipe books are fun and useful rewards, or subscribe to light recipe magazines such as *Cooking Light* or *Eating Well.* Magazines are a great value because the advertisers pay for most of the magazine's cost for you. Most magazines will gladly give you your first issue free.

952. *Give yourself a gold star.* Remember how much you enjoyed receiving a gold star when you did well in grade school? Try rewarding yourself as an adult with the same gold stars. List your goals and post them in your kitchen where you can see them each day. Whenever you achieve one of your goals, place a gold star by it. Now, whenever you walk by, you'll see your gold stars and be reminded that you really are finally doing it.

953. *Pay yourself.* Write yourself a check.

954. *Use exchange rewards.* Give yourself tokens, poker chips, or play money and then, when you have enough, exchange them for a nonfood reward.

955. *Learn something new.* Learn how to scuba dive, sew, knit, play the guitar, paint, garden, or photograph. The more activities you have that you enjoy, the less likely you are to get bored with life and binge. Learn with a friend and double the fun. Again, try to learn something that will directly help your weight loss. Take a weight-training class if you enjoy lifting weights, or a bike repair course if you enjoy biking.

956. *Do yourself over and have a blast.* Do something wacky for the new you and go have your hair and nails done as you've never done them before. Transform yourself from a flaming curly redhead one month into a straight-haired blond the next.

957. *Hot-oil massage.* Probably the only reward that will ever replace a hot fudge sundae is a hot-oil massage. Keep several scented oils handy and practice giving and receiving massage for stress control in particular. The most common method is called Swedish massage. This kind of massage relies heavily on five basic strokes:

- Tapotement. This is the familiar karate-chop stroke where the masseur taps, cups, or hacks you with the sides of the hands or fingertips.
- Effleurage. These are long gliding strokes that help to relax tense muscles and increase your circulation.
- Friction. This stroke involves the use of a circular and rolling motion on the muscle near the spine and the joints. It's a much more localized stroke than the others.
- Petrassage. This stroke kneads and squeezes the muscles.
- Vibration. To do this, tap rapidly with two fingers on one spot, or a series of spots.

The best way to receive a massage is nude. Clothing will only impede a massage. It also works best to lie flat on a hard table. Focus on relaxing your entire body during a massage and, when it's over, just lie still for a while with your eyes closed and enjoy your totally relaxed body.

958. **Form a partnership.** You may want to enlist the support of a partner, if you think you have a friend or spouse that would work. Your partner can be either thin or overweight, trying to lose weight or not trying to lose weight. What's important, among other things, is that you know you can count on your partner to be there when you need him or her. As you review your list of potential partners, make sure the person isn't overly critical about your weight, is easy to talk to about your weight, supports your food choices, is sincerely interested in helping you, won't become jealous, would be easy to speak to honestly even if you started to fail, would always be there for you, and can understand your weight problem.

Once you select a partner, set aside some time to sit down to discuss how you want your partner to help you. You can ask your partner to call once a day, week, or month to see how you're doing. He or she can praise and reward you with nonfood rewards or simply a few nice words, or be there when you step on the scale. Your partner can do everything that you're doing so that you both feel as if you're in this together. You both can exercise, shop for low-fat foods, learn to cook, learn new fitness activities, eat out, and so forth. Your partner can also give you a periodic reality check by reviewing your records to ensure you're where you're supposed to be. Partnerships help in some cases and in others have no effect. If you think you're the kind of person who could work well with a partner, then give it a try. If you'd rather go solo, then that's fine as well.

959. **Join a group.** If you enjoy working with groups of people in other areas of your life, then a group may help you to control your weight better. A group can brainstorm to help particular members solve problems, share similar experiences, and provide encouragement and support. Three good formal support groups are Overeaters Anonymous, TOPS (Take Off Pounds Sensibly), and Weight Watchers. Other options may include groups at your local hospital, health club, or church. You may also want to band together with people you know and start your own support group. If you do start a group, be sure to cultivate a spirit of cooperation among your members. During your first meetings, also keep in mind the guidelines in Tips 960 through 964 for good group behavior:

960. *Everyone should make a sincere effort to attend meetings and show up on time.*

961. *You don't have to talk all the time, but if you do have something to say, be sure to speak up.*

962. *Tune in to what other people are saying.* Listen to them, look them in the eyes, and acknowledge their statements.

963. *Avoid boredom by becoming involved with what the other person is saying.*

964. *Be sure everyone has an opportunity to voice comments, and above all, be very supportive of one another.*

965. **Sleep through late-night bingeing.** It's 1:00 A.M., it's been more than an hour since you tried counting sheep to fall asleep, and now the sheep have turned into slices of cold pizza washed down with fruit juice. You roll over and your spouse is sleeping like a rock. You stare at the ceiling some more and then, in utter despair, head for the fridge for a late-night snack and some late-night television. You then have trouble waking up in the morning, catnap all day long, and set yourself up for another night of insomnia. Sound familiar? If so, Tips 966 through 978 may help you sleep better and therefore binge less at night:

966. *You shouldn't try to sleep.* One of the worst things you can do is deliberately try to sleep. That's one way to make sure you'll stay awake all night. For many people reading works well. Think to yourself, "I'm not going to try to sleep; I'm going to read." There's nothing like a good book to help you take your mind off your troubles and tire your brain so that you can fall asleep.

967. *Avoid vigorous activity late at night.* Vigorous exercise can make you alert so that you can stay awake even longer.

968. *Sex usually doesn't work.* You may only fall asleep momentarily and then wake up again. As with vigorous exercise, it can awaken your body too much.

969. *Avoid alcohol.* Drinking alcohol will indeed knock you out for several hours. When you wake up to go to the bathroom, however, you may never fall back to sleep.

970. *Try relaxation techniques.* Most of these techniques are fancy names for the same thing. What it all boils down to is deep breathing and relaxed imagery. Take slow deep breaths and tell yourself

to relax. Then try to place relaxing pictures in your mind. Listen to, and focus on, your breathing. The sound of your breath is a natural relaxant.

971. *Take a hot bath.* A long, hot bath an hour or so before bed does wonders for sleep. It relaxes your muscles so that you can sleep peacefully throughout the night.

972. *Exercise three or four hours before bed.* Exercising during the day or in the evening works well. Try aerobic exercises such as walking, cycling, or swimming that work your muscles gently over a long period of time. Follow this workout with dinner, a hot bath, and a good book, and you're out like a light.

973. *Stay away from your bed and bedroom during the day.* Reading or lounging in bed during the day makes it difficult to sleep at night.

974. *If it's not working, then leave.* If you felt sleepy and went to bed, but then couldn't sleep, try going into another room for a while and then returning to bed.

975. *Wake up at the same time and go to bed at the same time every day.* It's important to establish a sleeping rhythm for your body. Setting a schedule and sticking to it as best you can will do this for you.

976. *Of course, you shouldn't nap during the day.*

977. *If your stomach growls at night, then try keeping a slice of apple or orange and a glass of water near your bed.*

978. *If you can't beat it, then make the most of your time.* If you try everything and fail, then admit you just need less sleep than most people and try to find pleasant activities to fill your extra hours.

979. **Use evening exercise to stop night eating:** To avoid eating late at night, try exercising in the evening at about 7:00 P.M. Join a health club with indoor facilities so that you can work out whenever you

want. The results may surprise you. Working out in the evening can do three positive things for you. First, it can get you out of the house and away from all of the house problems, which can grate on you and make you depressed. Second, it can make you feel so good about yourself that you won't want to pollute your healthy body with high-fat foods when you come home. Third, it can make you tired so that when you come home you fall right to sleep.

980. **Cope with frustration and reduce your stress.** Stress is a major cause of bingeing, and frustration is a major cause of stress. Tips 981 to 985 are strategies that will help you cope better with frustration and reduce your stress:

981. *Work hard at forgetting about past frustrations that led to failure.* It may help to slap your thigh or wrist, or put a rubber band around your wrist and snap it each time you catch yourself dwelling on a past frustration.

982. *Discover recurring patterns.* Look for patterns of frustration that you consistently experience. Discovering the pattern is the first major step toward eliminating it. For example, if you never got along well with your father, if you think your boss is a complete jerk, and if you think all elected officials are terrible, then you might have a pattern of frustration that stems from a problem with authority figures. Once you've identified a pattern, put together a list of three or so coping strategies you think might help. For instance, you could soothe yourself with a simple internal phrase, go for a walk, talk to a friend, or use the relaxed breathing strategy in tip 983 next time you're mad at your boss.

983. *Relaxation techniques.* If a wide variety of things constantly irritate you, consider trying a number of relaxation techniques. For example, you were speeding to get through a long red light, just missed it, and are now stuck at the light. Immediately take your eyes off the light, focus on the clouds or something pleasant, take several deep breaths, and exhale slowly with each one.

984. *Change it.* Stop and think for a moment why you're frustrated and then, if possible, avoid the cause in the future. For example, your kids won't ever eat spinach. Stop being so stubborn and feed them sweet peas. Maybe a particular traffic intersection annoys you. Take an alternate, possibly longer, but less stressful route.

985. *Roll with the punches.* Accept the fact that frustration is a part of the cost you pay to accomplish your goals. Things don't always go your way, you know that, so don't expect them to.

986. **Place goal photos on cupboards and the fridge.** This is a classic strategy to prevent overeating. What you want to avoid, however, is using fat pictures. Avoiding using pictures of what you don't want to be, and instead use beautiful pictures of what you want to become. Have small duplicates made of an older photo of you when you looked your best, or of someone you want to look like. Then place these on the fridge, by the goodie cupboard handle, and in your wallet and checkbook. Now whenever you feel like bingeing, you'll have a photo of your goal defending all the areas you would have to go through to binge.

987. **Don't blame the holidays.** It's not the holidays themselves that make you fat—it's how you respond to the holiday season that slaps the pounds on. Understand it's okay to break with tradition. You don't have to bake sugary sweet potatoes, turkey and fatty dressing, mashed potatoes and gravy, and desserts galore to be a good father, daughter-in-law, or wife during the holidays. Fix salmon, pasta, or light versions of traditional favorites. *Cooking Light* magazine's holiday editions can be helpful. They're always packed with tasty and manageable light recipes. Cook whatever you want and take control of the holiday season.

988. **Use HALT to identify what's causing your binge quickly.** As I'm sure you know, getting to the cause of your binge quickly is critical in order to deal with it effectively. Next time you're about to binge, remember the acronym HALT. HALT stands for Hunger—Anger—Loneliness—Tiredness. Of course there are a number of

reasons people binge, but these are typically among the most common. Next time you feel like bingeing remember HALT, and see if any of these reasons apply to you. Once you know the cause of your binge, you've taken the first step toward curing it fast.

989. **Slow your binge with sour tastes or nail polish.** Here are two tips designed to slow down your binge so that you can figure out its cause before it happens:
   • *Sour tastes.* When you feel as if you're about to binge, grab either a dill pickle, a lime, or a lemon and start to suck on it. While sucking on something sour, sit down at a table with some nice music in the background, take out a paper and pencil, and try to figure out your problem.
   • *Nail polish.* Take our your favorite color, or something wacky, and put two coats of nail polish on your nails. You can work on what's causing your binge while the polish dries.

990. **Put yourself in control.** Voluminous research suggests having a sense that you're in control of your life is one of the most important factors in determining your activity level, happiness, and health, and in some cases even how long you'll live! A good way to increase your sense of control over your world is to do aerobic exercise. In other words, just go for a walk, a jog, or a swim, or engage in in-line skating, cross-country skiing, or mountain biking. The result? You'll feel less anxious and more relaxed, and will have increased your sense of control over your own health and well-being.

991. **Never test your willpower.** Don't become arrogant and test your willpower by baking a double-chocolate fudge cake and then setting it on the counter. You're just asking for trouble.

992. **Burn calories while you watch television.** It's a fact that people who watch TV are more likely to be overweight than people who don't. So, obviously you should avoid the TV if you can. If you must watch TV, however, try exercising during the commercials.

You'll receive the benefits of exercise and you'll avoid commercials. A commercial break usually lasts about three minutes. This may not seem very long, but over the course of several shows it can really add up. Just hop on and off a cross-country ski machine or exercise bike, do push-ups, do sit-ups, or whatever. During the winter months you may even save a bit of money on your heating bill, since you'll need to keep the house cool for your "hot" body!

993. **Walk instead of eating candy when you're tired.** When you're tired, don't eat candy for energy. Research at California State University, Long Beach, demonstrates that while candy can boost your energy for 30 minutes after you consume it, one or two hours later your energy could be much lower than when you started. A 10-minute walk, however, can not only provide a huge energy boost in the first 30 minutes after the walk, but also keep your energy levels high for two hours after the walk. Ignore candy commercials and take a 10-minute brisk walk next time you want to energize yourself.

994. **Try not to punish yourself after you lapse.** A lapse is a slipup such as eating lots of a high-fat dessert. Almost everyone experiences highs and lows during weight control. The real issue isn't so much whether lapses will happen, but rather how you *respond* when they do happen. For instance, it's common for people to respond to a lapse by punishing themselves through deprivation. They may not let themselves eat for the rest of the day after lapsing in the morning, or they swear they'll never eat another bite of ice cream again after eating an entire pint. This will only set you up for another lapse. The one sure way to make yourself really want something is to tell yourself you can never have it. You may end up creating a behavior pattern of lapse, denial, lapse again, more denial, and lapse yet again. This terrible cycle can be avoided by not practicing denial or any other sort of punishment after a lapse. Instead, experiment with the ideas in Tips 995 through 1,000:

995. *Leave the situation that made you lapse.* Leave your home or office to escape the environment in which you experienced depression, boredom, anxiety, or frustration. Do this even if it's for only a few minutes.

996. *Remind yourself of how far you've come with your weight control.* You have made some progress and feel good about it. You don't want to continue to lapse and destroy what you've accomplished.

997. *Analyze your situation.* What put you at risk? Was it certain people, foods, or feelings? How can you avoid these negative factors next time? Transform your negative lapse into a positive learning experience.

998. *Don't wait; take charge immediately.* Once you've started to understand why you lapsed, take action right away. Have someone else clear away the rest of the food from the dinner table. Give away the rest of your cookies. Go meet a friend for tea. Go to a health club or for a long walk. Take action!

999. *Ask someone for help.* Ask friends and family if you can talk to them about how you're feeling. They can be a tremendous help. Just make certain you're completely honest with yourself and with them.

1,000. *Perhaps most important, remember that a lapse is* temporary! Experiencing a lapse doesn't mean you've destroyed your entire weight-control program. Try to keep looking at the big picture and remind yourself that you do many things throughout the day and week to control your weight. That one candy bar, piece of cake, or hot fudge sundae is just a drop in the bucket.

1,001. **Relax every muscle in your body to cope with stress.** Try this technique next time you're overwhelmed with stress for relief in about five minutes. Lie down flat, close your eyes, and take several deep and relaxing breaths. Now focus on one muscle group—say, your right forearm. Tense this muscle group for five seconds by making a fist, and then let it relax for 30 seconds. Now do the same thing to your left forearm. Next do it to your quads (your big thigh muscles), calves, neck, biceps (the large round muscle group on the front of your upper arm), bottom, shoulders, abdomen—all of your major muscle groups— one at a time until you've relaxed your entire body. With practice you'll learn which muscles tend to hold the most tension, and be able to use this tip to relax your trouble spot(s) quickly.

Afterword

Browse through this book several times. Write in it; copy from it; scribble in it; doodle in it; spill tea on the cover; use it! Refer to this book whenever you start a weight-control program or whenever you're having trouble with a weight-control program. Refer to it now and a year from now. Refer to it when you're young and when you're old, when you're fit and when you're fat. Refer to it when your life is going great, and refer to it when you feel as if your world is collapsing in all around you. The great thing about *1001 Simple Ways to Lose Weight* is that it contains so much useful information from such a wide variety of sources that, no matter what your situation is, you're bound to find something valuable every time you read it.

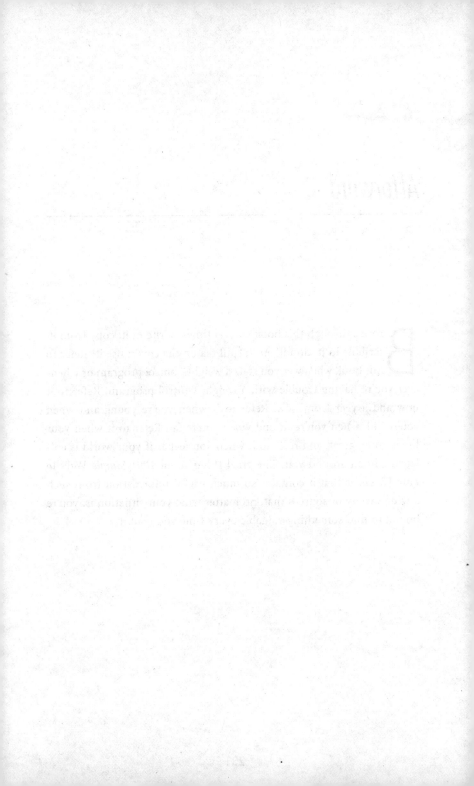

Appendix A

The Real-Life Menu Exchange

Sick and tired of diet books that proclaim you can eat more and weigh less, as long as it's bread, fish, or celery? Oh, and let's not forget all those scrumptious "free foods" such as all-you-can-eat bouillon, water, lemon juice, or cabbage. Are you bewildered by the thousands of new low-fat foods available? How do you know which taste good and are truly healthy or which taste bad and could jeopardize your health? Wouldn't it be great if you could afford to pay an expert staff to find the best-tasting and healthiest low-fat foods, and then to create a lifestyle food plan for you that used those foods? I wonder what it would cost—perhaps five to ten thousand dollars?

How about the price of this book! The Seattle Institute spent months walking up and down miles of supermarket aisles, checking ingredients and taste-testing every low-fat food we could find. After much dedicated snacking, we managed to identify a handful of amazing low-fat foods that taste as good as the high-fat originals but are healthier. We then combined our favorite low-fat foods with outstanding fast and flavorful low-fat recipes. The result is the Real-Life Menu Exchange. It's a practical lifestyle food plan specifically designed for everyday life. It's easy to follow, with no calorie or fat-gram counting, and since it's a menu exchange, any daily menu can be switched with any other daily menu. What's more, this plan is formulated according to the very latest scientific research so that you can lose weight as quickly as possible (one to two pounds per week) without jeopardizing good health and proper nutrition. You should in fact lose several pounds the first week alone. This will be primarily water weight, but it can be very exciting and possibly will motivate you to continue. After a week or two your weight loss should slow down to the healthy rate of one to two pounds a week as you start to rid yourself of more and more fat. You can follow this plan exactly, or, in combination with Steps 2 and 3 in Part I of this book, use it as a foundation on which to build your own eating plan.

In *Obesity: Theory and Therapy*, renowned weight-control expert Thomas Wadden, Ph.D., professor of psychology at Syracuse University, states he feels a nutritionally sound eating plan of 1,200 to 1,500 calories is a good starting place for many people wanting to control their weight. True lifestyle eating plans that incorporate a large variety of healthy foods you would normally eat, and don't severely restrict your calorie intake below 1,200 calories, can be an effective means to lose weight. As stated in the introduction to *1001 Simple Ways to Lose Weight*, however, to lose weight *and keep it off*, at some point you have to eliminate your bad habits and gain good ones through small changes you can manage in your day-to-day life. You can make these lifestyle changes before you lose weight, while you're losing it, or immediately after you've lost it. What matters is that you make them. You must change your habits if you want to ensure success over the long term. Once you've established your eating plan, review Steps 1 through 4 and Step 7 in Part I, and focus on eliminating any bad habits you might still have through small changes. If you do this, you'll have done much to ensure you'll finally lose your weight forever.

Getting Started

Be sure to check with your physician before using this menu exchange if you have any medical problems. Children, teenagers, breast-feeding women, and pregnant women have special nutrition requirements and so should not use this menu exchange.

Each of the daily menus listed is approximately 1,200 to 1,300 calories. These are reasonable calorie levels for women to lose weight. If you're a man, just increase your food portions by 50 percent and consume two extra slices of whole-grain bread each day. This way couples and families won't have to prepare separate menus for men and women. Recipes for many of the dishes are in the "Recipes" section that follows the menus for Day 30.

After you've read the preceding information, you're ready to start using the menu exchange. Just be sure to:

- Begin increasing your physical activity by performing Steps 5 through 7 in Part I of this book. You could lose all your excess weight using this plan without doing any physical activity, but if you do so the chances are very good that you'll gain it back in two or three years. As I've stated throughout this book, if you want to lose weight and keep it off, you should exercise moderately on a regular basis by participating in an activity you enjoy.

- Don't cut any fat from this plan. It's carefully structured so that you'll receive approximately 15 to 20 percent of your calories from fat. This is a reasonable fat intake level for good health and weight loss.

- Pay attention to the wording in the daily menus. For instance, if a menu suggests using "lower-fat" margarine, then check the label of your margarine to make sure it's "lower fat" instead of "fat free." If a menu calls for "light" mayonnaise, use it instead of "fat free."

- Drink six to eight cups of noncaffeinated liquids each day. You can drink caffeinated liquids in moderation but, because they're diuretics, they don't count toward your daily fluid requirement.

- Plan your meals at least one day in advance.

- Shop from a grocery list so that the foods the menu plan requires are handy.

- Don't be afraid to experiment with new foods.

- If you have leftovers to use up—such as chicken—find a daily menu with that ingredient in it, and use it the next day instead of proceeding through the menus in order.

- Limit consumption of egg yolks to no more than four per week from all sources.

- Weigh and measure your food if you're at all unsure about a portion size.

Daily Menus[10]

Day 1

Breakfast

Two frozen fat-free waffles topped with 1 cup sliced fresh strawberries or peaches dusted with 1 tablespoon powdered sugar; 1 cup skim milk.

Lunch

Turkey Sandwich with Chips: 2 ounces low-fat turkey breast, two regular slices whole-grain bread (not to exceed 70 calories and 1 gram of fat per slice), 1 tablespoon low-fat mayonnaise mixed with a dash of Dijon-style mustard or ketchup, half of a sliced fresh tomato or four to six slices fresh cucumber, freshly ground pepper to taste; 11 low-fat potato chips (serving should not exceed 2 grams of fat and 60 calories); one yellow or red bell pepper cut into strips.

[10]Serving size and number in Appendixes A and B are based on the American Dietetic and American Diabetes Associations' "Exchange Lists for Weight Management," and on the U.S. Department of Agriculture/U.S. Department of Health and Human Services' "Food Guide Pyramid."

Snack (anytime)

Double Chocolate Swirl: 12 chocolate Teddy Grahams (teddy bear cookies) dipped in one container fat-free chocolate pudding. If you don't like chocolate, try substituting one container vanilla fat-free pudding.

Dinner

Beef Tenderloin with Peppercorns (see page 259); ½ cup boiled red or new potatoes seasoned with your choice of Mrs. Dash or other prepared seasoning and 1 tablespoon Fleischmann's 5 Calorie Butter Spread; ½ cup steamed fresh cauliflower or broccoli topped with 1 tablespoon Fleischmann's 10 Calorie Cheddar Cheese Spread; 1 cup skim milk; one orange.

Day 2

Breakfast

Three-quarters cup dry high-fiber cereal (choose from Healthy Options Food List in Step 2); 1 cup skim milk; ½ cup orange or grapefruit juice.

Lunch

Ham Sandwich with Cheese Crackers: 2 ounces Canadian bacon, 2 regular slices whole-grain bread, 1 tablespoon low-fat mayonnaise mixed with a dash of Dijon-style mustard or ketchup, half of a sliced fresh tomato or four to six slices fresh cucumber, freshly ground pepper to taste; 32 Nabisco SnackWell's Zesty Cheese Crackers; 1 cup skim milk.

Snack (anytime)

Fruit in Pudding: Dip the tips of 1 cup whole strawberries or seven dried apricot halves into one container fat-free chocolate pudding, then eat remaining pudding.

Dinner

One serving Zesty Scallops (see page 260); ½ cup boiled red or new potatoes seasoned with your choice of Mrs. Dash or other prepared seasoning and 1 tablespoon lower-fat tub margarine; ½ cup steamed cauliflower or broccoli salted and peppered to taste.

Day 3

Breakfast

Three-quarters cup dry high-fiber cereal; 1 ounce Canadian bacon; 1 cup skim milk; half of a banana by itself or sliced and added to cereal. [Read lunch recipe, prepare quick tuna mixture, and refrigerate either at home or when you get to work.]

Lunch

One serving Easy Tuna Pocket with Lemon and Basil (see page 261); two plums or one tangerine.

Snack (anytime)

One-half cup Dannon frozen yogurt.

Dinner

One Mex Burrito (see page 261); ½ cup cooked brown rice;
2 cups tossed salad topped with 2 tablespoons commercial
fat-free salad dressing (to liven up your salads, see Tips 223
through 251); two servings Honeydew-Heaven Slush
(Tip 385).

Day 4

Breakfast

One whole warm or toasted bagel halved and topped with
1 tablespoon lower-fat tub margarine; 1 cup skim milk.

Lunch

Bacon and Lettuce Sandwich: two slices turkey bacon,
two regular slices plain or toasted whole-grain bread,
1 tablespoon low-fat mayonnaise mixed with a dash of Dijon-
style mustard or ketchup, one lettuce leaf, half of a sliced
fresh tomato or four to six slices fresh cucumber, ¼ cup raw
bean sprouts (optional), freshly ground pepper to taste; one
orange; 1 cup skim milk.

Snack (anytime)

One single-stick frozen juice pop (not to exceed 30 calories).

Dinner

One serving Quick Poached Cod (see page 262); two servings
Nutty Rice Pilaf (see page 263); 2 cups tossed salad with
1 tablespoon plus 2 teaspoons fat-free salad dressing; ½ cup
mandarin oranges canned in juice.

Day 5

Breakfast

One whole English muffin; 1 tablespoon fruit jam; one slice turkey bacon; half of a grapefruit or one orange.

Lunch

Hot Ham and Cheese Pocket: Inside half of a 6-inch whole-grain pita pocket stuff 2 ounces Canadian bacon, 1 cup raw broccoli florets, and 2 ounces shredded reduced-fat mild cheddar cheese (not to exceed 90 calories per ounce). Microwave until cheese melts and broccoli is soft. If you don't have a microwave, steam broccoli first, then bake sandwich in oven until cheese melts. Serve with one Granny Smith or other apple.

Snack (anytime)

Stir 1 tablespoon chocolate minimorsels and 1 tablespoon crème de menthe into 1 cup Dannon vanilla nonfat yogurt.

Dinner

One serving Orange Pork Tenderloin (see page 263); Cinnamon Sweet Potato (see Tip 87); 1 cup steamed fresh or frozen green peas.

Day 6

Breakfast

One cup cooked oatmeal or other hot cereal; 1 cup skim milk; ¾ cup fresh berries.

Lunch

One and one-half servings Progresso Spicy Chicken and Penne Pasta soup with ½ cup cooked pasta added to soup; half of a sliced cucumber soaked for 5 minutes in balsamic vinegar.

Snack (anytime)

One cup fruit-flavored nonfat yogurt.

Dinner

One serving Black Beans with Sherry over Rice (see page 264); 2 cups tossed salad topped with 2 tablespoons fat-free salad dressing and either a sixth of a medium avocado, eight ripe olives, or 1½ teaspoons dry roasted sunflower seeds; 1¼ cups watermelon cubes or two plums.

Day 7

Breakfast

Three-quarters cup dry high-fiber cereal (choose from Healthy Options Food List in Step 2); 1 cup skim milk; half of a banana by itself or sliced and added to cereal.

Lunch

Toasted Ham and Cheese: Toast two regular slices whole-grain bread, top with 2 ounces Canadian bacon and three slices Kraft Fat-Free Singles, heat until cheese melts, arrange three or four thin tomato slices on top of melted cheese, and sprinkle with optional garlic powder; one medium raw carrot or stalk of celery.

Snack (anytime)

New Zealand Fruit Mix (Tip 96).

Dinner

One serving Sensational Sesame Chicken (Tip 405); 1 cup
boiled red or new potatoes seasoned with your choice of Mrs.
Dash or other prepared seasoning and 1 tablespoon lower-fat
tub margarine; ½ cup steamed fresh or frozen corn or peas;
one tangerine or orange.

Day 8

Breakfast

One serving Crazy Banana Pancakes (see page 265) topped with
1 tablespoon lower-fat tub margarine; half of a banana; 1 cup
skim milk.

Lunch

Turkey Sandwich with Chips: (see lunch for Day 1); one yellow
or red bell pepper cut into strips; 1 cup skim milk.

Snack (anytime)

Dip the tips of 1 cup whole strawberries or seven dried apricot
halves into 1 tablespoon Hershey's chocolate syrup.

Dinner

One serving Snappy Mexican Snapper (Tip 408); ½ cup boiled
red or new potatoes seasoned with your choice of Mrs. Dash

or other prepared seasoning and 2 teaspoons lower-fat tub margarine; ½ cup steamed fresh cauliflower or broccoli salted and peppered to taste.

Day 9

Breakfast

Two frozen fat-free waffles topped with ¾ cup fresh blackberries or blueberries or one sliced fresh peach, dusted with 1 tablespoon powdered sugar; 1 cup skim milk.

Lunch

Roast Beef or Honey Ham Sandwich: 2 ounces low-fat roast beef or honey ham luncheon meat, two regular slices whole-grain bread, 1 tablespoon plus 2 teaspoons low-fat mayonnaise mixed with a dash of Dijon-style mustard or ketchup, half of a sliced fresh tomato or four to six slices fresh cucumber, freshly ground pepper to taste; one medium raw carrot or stalk of celery.

Snack (anytime)

Sprinkle half of a grapefruit with ½ teaspoon brown sugar and ½ teaspoon apple-pie spice, then broil in oven until sugar melts.

Dinner

One serving Superb Sweet Chicken (Tip 411); one serving Fabulously Fragrant Rice (see page 266); ½ cup steamed frozen or fresh corn; 1 cup skim milk.

Day 10
Breakfast

One whole English muffin topped with 1 tablespoon lower-fat tub margarine; half of a grapefruit or one kiwi fruit. [Read dinner recipe and prepare quick marinade for dinner.]

Lunch

Mex Burrito (see page 261).

Snack (anytime)

One single-stick frozen juice pop (not to exceed 30 calories).

Dinner

One serving Quick Teriyaki Chicken (see page 266); ½ cup cooked regular long-grain rice; 1 cup small cantaloupe balls; 2 cups tossed salad with 2 tablespoons fat-free salad dressing.

Day 11
Breakfast

One whole warm or toasted bagel halved and topped with 1 tablespoon raspberry or other jam; 1 cup skim milk; one orange or nectarine. [Read lunch recipe, prepare tuna mixture, and refrigerate mixture either at home or when you get to work.]

Lunch

One serving Easy Tuna Pocket with Lemon and Basil (see page 261); two plums or one tangerine; 1 cup raw cauliflower florets plain or dipped in 1 tablespoon Dijon-style mustard.

Snack (anytime)

Two Nabisco SnackWell's Devil's Food Cookie Cakes. After you
open the stay-fresh package, store them in pairs (two cookie
cakes equal one serving) in zip-top sandwich bags out
of sight.

Dinner

One Granddaddy Pork Sandwich (see page 267); 11 low-fat
potato chips (serving should not exceed 2 grams of fat and
60 calories); 2 cups tossed salad with 2 tablespoons fat-free
salad dressing; 1 cup skim milk.

Day 12

Breakfast

One and one-half cups dry high-fiber cereal; 1 cup skim milk;
½ cup orange or grapefruit juice. [Read dinner recipe,
prepare quick marinade, and refrigerate meat in marinade for
dinner.]

Lunch

Pita Pizzazz: Toss 2 ounces low-fat turkey breast, ½ cup
garbanzo (chickpeas) or other beans, half of a sliced tomato,
and 1 cup salad greens with 2 tablespoons fat-free salad
dressing, then stuff into half of a 6-inch whole-grain pita
pocket.

Snack (anytime)

Twelve Keebler Wheatables.

Dinner

One serving London Broil (see page 268); one small baked
potato topped with 1 tablespoon Fleischmann's 5 Calorie
Butter Spread and your choice of Mrs. Dash or other
prepared seasoning; ½ cup steamed asparagus or broccoli
topped with 2 ounces shredded reduced-fat mild cheddar
cheese (no more than 90 calories per ounce); one orange.

Day 13

Breakfast

One whole English muffin topped with 1 tablespoon lower-fat
tub margarine; half of a grapefruit or banana; 1 cup skim
milk.

Lunch

Chef Salad: 2 cups lettuce, 2 ounces chopped low-fat turkey
breast, half of a sliced tomato, half of a sliced cucumber,
one-quarter of a chopped yellow bell pepper, six or so thin
carrot shavings using a vegetable peeler, ½ cup bean sprouts,
2 tablespoons fat-free Italian salad dressing; two slices toasted
French bread topped with 1 tablespoon lower-fat tub
margarine and optional garlic powder.

Snack (anytime)

Combine 1 tablespoon orange marmalade with 1 cup vanilla
nonfat yogurt, one sliced fresh peach, and a dash of
cinnamon.

Dinner

One serving Orange Pork Tenderloin (see page 263);
Cinnamon Sweet Potato (Tip 87); ½ cup steamed frozen or
fresh green peas.

Day 14

Breakfast

One poached egg; half of a bagel topped with 1 tablespoon
lower-fat tub margarine; ½ cup vanilla nonfat yogurt.

Lunch

Toasted Ham and Cheese (see lunch for Day 7); one
medium raw carrot or stalk of celery; one Granny Smith or
other apple.

Snack (anytime)

Ten gourmet jelly beans (see Tip 65).

Dinner

Italian Delight: 1 cup cooked spaghetti, 1 cup sliced fresh
mushrooms, 1¼ cups steamed broccoli, ¾ cup spaghetti
sauce (no more than 75 calories), 2 tablespoons grated
Parmesan cheese; one slice French bread topped with
1 tablespoon Fleischmann's 5 Calorie Butter Spread, a
sprinkling of garlic powder, a pinch of basil, then toasted;
15 grapes.

Day 15

Breakfast

Two frozen fat-free waffles topped with 1 cup sliced fresh strawberries or peaches dusted with 1 tablespoon powdered sugar; 1 cup skim milk. [Read dinner recipe and place chicken in quick and easy marinade, then refrigerate.]

Lunch

Pastrami or Smoked Ham Sandwich with Crackers (see lunch for Day 1, but substitute low-fat pastrami or smoked ham luncheon meat); 27 Keebler Wheatables; one medium raw carrot or stalk of celery.

Snack (anytime)

Two Nabisco SnackWell's Devil's Food Cookie Cakes; 1 cup skim milk.

Dinner

One serving Outrageous Chicken Sandwich (see page 268); one yellow or red bell pepper cut into strips; ⅓ cup pineapple canned in its own juice or ¾ cup raw pineapple.

Day 16

Breakfast

One whole warm or toasted bagel halved and topped with 1 tablespoon lower-fat tub margarine and 1 tablespoon strawberry or other fruit jam; 1 cup skim milk.

Lunch

Two servings Progresso Hearty Chicken Soup with ½ cup cooked spiral pasta added to soup; one medium raw carrot or stalk of celery.

Snack (anytime)

Banana Blitz: In blender combine half of a banana, 1 cup skim milk, ½ teaspoon vanilla, sugar-free sweetener to taste, and several ice cubes. Blend until smooth.

Dinner

One serving Quick Poached Cod (see page 262); two servings Nutty Rice Pilaf (see page 263); 2 cups tossed salad with 2 tablespoons fat-free salad dressing; one pear or two plums.

Day 17

Breakfast

One serving Crazy Banana Pancakes (see page 265); half of a banana; 1 cup skim milk.

Lunch

Pita Pizzazz (see lunch for Day 12).

Snack (anytime)

Stir 1 tablespoon chocolate minimorsels and 1 tablespoon crème de menthe into 1 cup vanilla nonfat yogurt.

Dinner

Beef Tenderloin with Peppercorns (see page 259); ½ cup boiled red or new potatoes seasoned with your choice of prepared seasoning and 1 tablespoon Fleischmann's 5 Calorie Butter Spread; ½ cup steamed fresh cauliflower or broccoli topped with 1 tablespoon Fleischmann's 10 Calorie Cheddar Cheese Spread; 1 cup skim milk; one orange.

Day 18

Breakfast

Two frozen fat-free waffles topped with 1 cup sliced fresh strawberries or peaches dusted with 1 tablespoon powdered sugar; 1 cup skim milk.

Lunch

Bacon and Lettuce Sandwich (see lunch for Day 4).

Snack (anytime)

Combine 1 teaspoon orange marmalade with ½ cup vanilla nonfat yogurt, 1 sliced fresh peach, and a dash of cinnamon; 12 Keebler Wheatables.

Dinner

Turkey Cheese Loaf (see page 269); one small baked potato topped with 1 tablespoon Fleischmann's 5 Calorie Butter Spread and your choice of Mrs. Dash or other prepared seasoning; 1 cup steamed asparagus or broccoli topped with 1 ounce reduced-fat mild cheddar cheese (not to exceed 90 calories per ounce).

Day 19

Breakfast

One bagel topped with 1 tablespoon lower-fat tub margarine; half of a grapefruit or one kiwi fruit; 1½ cups skim milk.

Lunch

Turkey Sandwich with Chips (see lunch for Day 1); one yellow or red bell pepper cut into strips.

Snack (anytime)

One single-stick frozen juice pop (not to exceed 30 calories).

Dinner

One serving Orange and Clove Snapper (see page 270); two servings Savory Rice (see page 271); ½ cup cooked carrots; ½ cup steamed pea pods topped with 1 tablespoon lower-fat tub margarine; two plums or one peach.

Day 20

Breakfast

One cup cooked oatmeal or other hot cereal; 1 cup skim milk; in cereal you can put 1 tablespoon raisins or ¾ cup fresh berries.

Lunch

Chef Salad with French bread (see lunch for Day 13).

Snack (anytime)

Combine 1 tablespoon orange marmalade with 1 cup vanilla nonfat yogurt, one sliced fresh peach, and a dash of cinnamon.

Dinner

One serving San Diego Oven-Fried Chicken (Tip 344); ½ cup steamed fresh or frozen corn; ½ cup cooked brown rice; one orange.

Day 21

Breakfast

One whole warm or toasted bagel halved and topped with 1 tablespoon lower-fat tub margarine; 1 cup skim milk.

Lunch

Bacon and Lettuce Sandwich (see lunch for Day 4): one golden delicious or other apple.

Snack (anytime)

Two Nabisco Fat-Free SnackWell's Devil's Food Cookie Cakes; 1 cup skim milk.

Dinner

One serving London Broil (see page 268); one small baked potato seasoned with 1 tablespoon lower-fat tub margarine and your choice of Mrs. Dash or other prepared seasoning; ½ cup steamed asparagus or broccoli; 2 cups tossed salad with 2 tablespoons fat-free salad dressing; one orange or nectarine.

Day 22

Breakfast

One and one-half cups dry high-fiber cereal (choose from Healthy Options Food List in Step 2); 1 cup skim milk; 15 red or green grapes. [Read lunch recipe, prepare quick tuna mixture, and refrigerate mixture either at home or when you get to work.]

Lunch

One serving Easy Tuna Pocket with Lemon and Basil (see page 261); 1 cup raw cauliflower plain or dipped in Dijon-style mustard.

Snack (anytime)

One Milky Way Light candy bar.

Dinner

One serving Superb Sweet Chicken (Tip 411); one serving Fabulously Fragrant Rice (see page 266); 1 cup raw or ½ cup steamed pea pods; 1 cup vanilla nonfat yogurt mixed with 1 cup sliced strawberries or other berry of choice.

Day 23

Breakfast

One poached egg; one slice turkey bacon; half of an English muffin topped with 1 tablespoon strawberry or other jam; half of a grapefruit or one kiwi fruit.

Lunch

Sandwich with Cheese Crackers: 1 ounce or about three slices low-fat luncheon meat, two regular slices whole-grain bread, 1 tablespoon low-fat mayonnaise mixed with a dash of Dijon-style mustard or ketchup, one lettuce leaf, half of a sliced fresh tomato or four to six slices fresh cucumber, freshly ground pepper to taste; 16 Nabisco SnackWell's Zesty Cheese Reduced Fat Crackers or other crackers (serving not to exceed 60 calories and 1 gram of fat); one red delicious or other apple; one medium raw or ½ cup cooked carrot.

Snack (anytime)

Banana Blitz (see snack for Day 16).

Dinner

Couscous Casserole (see page 271); 1 cup raw or ½ cup steamed pea pods; 15 red or green grapes; ¾ cup skim milk.

Day 24

Breakfast

One poached egg; one English muffin topped with 1 tablespoon lower-fat tub margarine; 1 cup skim milk.

Lunch

Pita Pizzazz (see lunch for Day 12).

Snack (anytime)

Sprinkle half of a grapefruit with ½ teaspoon brown sugar and ½ teaspoon apple-pie spice, then broil in oven until sugar melts.

Dinner

Italian Delight (see dinner for Day 14).

Day 25

Breakfast

One cup cooked oatmeal or other hot cereal; 1 cup skim milk; ¾ cup fresh berries.

Lunch

Chef Salad with French bread (see lunch for Day 13).

Snack (anytime)

One cup Dannon frozen yogurt.

Dinner

One serving Shrimp Festival (see page 272); one serving Savory Rice (see page 271); ½ cup steamed fresh or frozen peas; 1 cup small honeydew melon balls.

Day 26

Breakfast

One serving Crazy Banana Pancakes (see page 265) topped with
1 tablespoon lower-fat tub margarine; half of a banana;
1½ cups skim milk.

Lunch

Two servings Progresso Hearty Chicken Soup with ½ cup
cooked spiral pasta added to soup; one golden delicious or
other apple.

Snack (anytime)

One serving South Pacific Cantaloupe Salad: Combine ¾ cup
vanilla nonfat yogurt with 1 teaspoon fresh lime juice and
½ teaspoon nutmeg. Using the small end of a melon baller,
ball one fresh cantaloupe. Combine yogurt mixture with
cantaloupe balls and serve. One serving equals 1 cup.

Dinner

One serving Quick Poached Cod (see page 262); one serving
Nutty Rice Pilaf (see page 263); 2 cups tossed salad with
2 tablespoons fat-free salad dressing.

Day 27

Breakfast

One whole English muffin; 1 tablespoon lower-fat tub
margarine; half of a grapefruit or one pear; 1 cup skim milk.

Lunch

Broccoli and Pasta Salad: Toss 1 cup steamed firm broccoli,
1 cup cooked pasta, ½ cup chopped tomato, and chopped
fresh basil to taste with 2 tablespoons fat-free Italian dressing.

Snack (anytime)

One container prepared fat-free pudding.

Dinner

One serving Orange-Lemon Game Hen (see page 273); 1 cup
boiled red or new potatoes seasoned with your choice of
Mrs. Dash or other prepared seasoning and topped with ½
cup or 2 ounces fat-free mild cheddar cheese; ½ cup steamed
carrots; one sliced orange.

Day 28

Breakfast

Half of a bagel topped with 1 tablespoon lower-fat tub
margarine; 1 cup skim milk.

Lunch

Roast Beef or Pastrami Sandwich with Chips: 2 ounces low-fat
roast beef or pastrami luncheon meat, two regular slices
whole-grain bread, 2 tablespoons fat-free salad dressing or
Dijon mustard, half of a sliced fresh tomato or four to six
slices fresh cucumber, freshly ground pepper to taste; 18
Mother's Potato Snaps; one medium raw carrot or stalk
of celery.

Snack (anytime)

One cup vanilla nonfat yogurt mixed with ¾ cup fresh berries.

Dinner

Beef Tenderloin with Peppercorns (see page 259); one small
potato seasoned with your choice of prepared seasoning and
1 tablespoon Fleischmann's 5 Calorie Butter Spread; 2 cups
tossed salad with 2 tablespoons fat-free salad dressing;
1¼ cups watermelon cubes or two plums.

Day 29

Breakfast

Three-quarters cup dry high-fiber cereal; 1 cup skim milk.

Lunch

One serving Healthy Choice Beef and Potato soup; one regular
slice toasted whole-grain bread topped with 1 tablespoon
lower-fat tub margarine and a sprinkling of garlic powder;
one red or yellow bell pepper cut into strips; one pear.

Snack (anytime)

Stir 1 tablespoon chocolate minimorsels and 2 tablespoons
crème de menthe into 1 cup vanilla nonfat yogurt.

Dinner

One serving Orange and Clove Snapper (see page 270); two
servings Savory Rice (see page 271); ½ cup cooked carrots;
¾ cup steamed pea pods topped with 1 tablespoon lower-fat
tub margarine; two plums or one peach.

Day 30

Breakfast

One whole warm or toasted bagel halved and topped with
1 tablespoon fruit jam; one slice turkey bacon; 1 cup skim
milk; one orange or nectarine. [Read dinner recipe and place
meat in quick and easy marinade.]

Lunch

Hot Ham and Cheese Pocket (see lunch for Day 5); serve with
one Granny Smith or other apple.

Snack (anytime)

Two Nabisco Fat-Free SnackWell's Devil's Food Cookie Cakes.

Dinner

One serving Outrageous Chicken Sandwich (see page 268);
18 Mother's Potato Snaps; one yellow or red bell pepper cut
into strips; ⅓ cup pineapple canned in its own juice or ¾ cup
raw pineapple.

Recipes for the Real-Life Menu Exchange

Beef Tenderloin with Peppercorns

1 pound 3 ounces beef tenderloin
1 clove garlic, cut lengthwise into slivers
2½ teaspoons olive oil
¼ teaspoon dried thyme
1½ teaspoons cracked black peppercorns
¼ teaspoon dried rosemary

¼ teaspoon dried sage
Salt to taste

1. Preheat oven to 425 degrees. Use a sharp knife to make small incisions in tenderloin, then insert a garlic sliver into each incision. Rub olive oil on tenderloin.

2. In a small bowl combine thyme, peppercorns, rosemary, and sage, then pat the mixture onto all sides of tenderloin.

3. Roast tenderloin in a small shallow roasting pan for 10 minutes, reduce heat to 350 degrees, and roast another 20 minutes for medium doneness. Salt to taste. Let cool 10 minutes before slicing.

Makes 5 servings with 210 calories and 12 grams fat each.

Zesty Scallops

2 tablespoons freshly squeezed lime juice
2 tablespoons freshly squeezed lemon juice
2 tablespoons dry white wine
2 teaspoons Tabasco
2 teaspoons olive oil
1 scallion, chopped
1 yellow bell pepper, sliced thin
1 green bell pepper, sliced thin
1 red bell pepper, sliced thin
1 pound bay scallops, rinsed and patted dry
1 teaspoon salt
1 tablespoon minced fresh basil *or* 1 teaspoon dried basil

1. In a small bowl mix together lime juice, lemon juice, white wine, and Tabasco. Set aside.

2. Heat olive oil over high heat in a large nonstick skillet, then add scallion and peppers and cook, stirring constantly, for 3 minutes. Add wine mixture and cook 1 minute more.

3. Stir in scallops, salt, and basil. Reduce heat to medium, cover, and cook for 3–4 minutes, or until scallops are opaque.

Makes 4 servings with 159 calories and 3 grams fat each.

Easy Tuna Pocket with Lemon and Basil

½ cup chopped celery
¼ cup sliced green onions
2 6½-ounce cans tuna packed in water, drained
2 tablespoons commercial oil-free Italian dressing
1 teaspoon olive oil
2 tablespoons lemon juice
¼ teaspoon low-sodium lemon-pepper seasoning
1 tablespoon water
1 clove garlic, minced
2 tablespoons chopped fresh basil
3 whole-grain pita bread rounds (6-inch), cut in half crosswise
6 slices fresh tomato about ¼ inch thick
6 leaves green-leaf lettuce

1. In a large bowl stir together the first three ingredients. In another bowl stir together the next seven ingredients and pour over the tuna mixture. Refrigerate covered for at least 1 hour.

2. Place one tomato slice and one lettuce leaf in each pita half, spoon in tuna mixture, and serve.

Makes 6 servings with 183 calories and 5.8 grams fat each.

Mex Burrito

½ cup Rosarita's vegetarian refried beans
1 whole-wheat tortilla
½ cup cooked brown rice
2 tablespoons Pace Thick & Chunky Salsa

2 ounces reduced-fat cheddar cheese, shredded
½ red bell pepper cut into thin strips
½ yellow bell pepper cut into thin strips

Preheat oven to 400 degrees. Spoon beans onto tortilla. Top with remaining ingredients. Roll tortilla into a tube, place on cookie sheet, and bake in oven until cheese melts.

Makes 1 serving with 492 calories and 12.8 grams fat.

Quick Poached Cod

1 cup 1-percent milk
4 cod fillets (5 ounces each)
1 tablespoon plus 1 teaspoon reduced-calorie tub margarine
3 tablespoons all-purpose flour
¼ cup chicken broth
½ teaspoon salt
¼ teaspoon freshly ground black pepper
2 tablespoons minced fresh parsley
4 sprigs fresh parsley

1. Heat milk in a skillet, add cod fillets, cover, and poach 4–5 minutes, or until fish flakes easily when tested with a fork. Transfer fish to a serving platter with a slotted spoon and set milk aside.

2. Melt margarine in a saucepan and gradually add flour. Cook about 2 minutes over low heat until bubbly. Remove from heat, whisk in chicken broth and hot milk, then add salt, pepper, and minced parsley. Return to low heat and cook about 3 minutes, or until sauce thickens, stirring constantly. Pour sauce over fish, and garnish with parsley sprigs.

Makes 4 servings with 183 calories and 4 grams fat each.

Nutty Rice Pilaf

1 clove garlic, minced
2 tablespoons minced onion
2 cups canned chicken broth
¼ cup raisins
1 cup basmati rice, uncooked
1 teaspoon reduced-calorie margarine
1 tablespoon minced walnuts

1. Coat a large saucepan with vegetable cooking spray and place over medium-high heat until hot. Add garlic and onion and sauté until tender. Pour in chicken broth, bring to boil, stir in raisins and rice, cover, reduce heat, and simmer for 15 minutes.

2. While rice is cooking, coat a large saucepan with vegetable cooking spray, add margarine, and place over medium-high heat until pan is hot. Add walnuts and cook, stirring constantly, until nuts are toasted. Set aside.

3. When rice is done cooking, remove from heat and let stand 10 minutes. Using a fork, gently toss walnuts and rice to combine and serve hot.

Makes 8 half-cup servings with 120 calories and 1.9 grams fat each.

Orange Pork Tenderloin

1½ tablespoons grainy (sometimes called "stone ground") prepared mustard
¼ teaspoon finely chopped fresh rosemary
1 clove garlic, minced
Pinch freshly ground black pepper
1 pound pork tenderloin

¼ cup low-sugar orange marmalade

½ cup water

¼ cup chicken broth

1. Preheat oven to 400 degrees. Stir together mustard, rosemary, garlic, and pepper in a small bowl. Make two or three cuts about halfway through the pork tenderloin running against the grain. Spread mustard mixture along the cuts, place on rack *above* a roasting pan, and brush with 2 tablespoons orange marmalade. Add water to roasting pan to prevent meat from drying. Bake for 40 to 45 minutes or until cooked through.

2. Simmer chicken broth and remaining marmalade in a small saucepan until thickened. Spoon over tenderloin and serve hot.

Makes 4 servings with 160 calories and 3 grams fat each.

Black Beans with Sherry over Rice

1 tablespoon plus 1 teaspoon olive oil

1 tablespoon finely chopped garlic

1 cup finely chopped green bell pepper

½ cup finely chopped yellow onion

1 15-ounce can black beans

1½ cups canned plum tomatoes, chopped coarse

½ cup water

1 cup chicken broth

1 tablespoon plus 1 teaspoon dry sherry

1 bay leaf

¼ teaspoon dried oregano

¼ teaspoon hot pepper sauce

½ teaspoon dried thyme

1 tablespoon chopped fresh cilantro

Salt and pepper to taste

4 cups cooked regular long-grain rice

1. Heat oil in a saucepan over medium-low heat, then add garlic, bell pepper, and onion. Sauté 15 minutes, stirring occasionally.

2. Add beans, tomatoes, water, chicken broth, sherry, bay leaf, oregano, hot pepper sauce, and thyme. Bring to a boil over high heat, then reduce heat and simmer, stirring occasionally, for 45 minutes, or until vegetables are tender and sauce thickens. You can add hot water if mixture becomes too thick. Stir in cilantro, season with salt and pepper to taste, remove bay leaf, and serve over rice.

Makes 4 servings with 507 calories and 6 grams fat each.

Crazy Banana Pancakes

1 cup nonfat buttermilk
1 teaspoon baking soda
½ cup frozen egg substitute, thawed
½ cup mashed ripe banana
1 tablespoon vegetable oil
1 cup all-purpose flour
⅛ teaspoon salt
1 tablespoon sugar

1. In a medium-sized bowl stir together buttermilk and baking soda, then add egg substitute, banana, and oil. In a large bowl combine flour, salt, and sugar, then make a well in center of mixture. Whisk buttermilk mixture and add to dry ingredients, stirring just until dry ingredients are moistened.

2. Spray a nonstick griddle with vegetable cooking spray and preheat to 350 degrees. Pour ¼ cup batter onto hot griddle for each pancake.

Makes 6 servings (two 4-inch pancakes) with 150 calories and 2.8 grams fat each.

Fabulously Fragrant Rice

2½ cups water
½ teaspoon salt
¼ teaspoon ground turmeric
¼ teaspoon ground cardamom
¼ teaspoon ground red pepper
⅛ teaspoon ground cinnamon
1¼ cups basmati rice
Dash saffron

In a medium saucepan combine all ingredients, bring to a boil, stir, reduce heat, cover, and simmer for 20 minutes. Remove from heat and let stand 10 minutes. Fluff with fork and serve hot.

Makes 8 half-cup servings with 117 calories and 0.2 gram fat each.

Quick Teryaki Chicken

¼ cup low-sodium soy sauce
3 tablespoons freshly squeezed orange juice
3 tablespoons light corn syrup
1 clove garlic, crushed
1 tablespoon dark brown sugar, firmly packed
½ teaspoon ground ginger
1½ pounds whole chicken breasts, skinned and split

1. Combine all ingredients except chicken in a bowl or jar with a tight-fitting lid, then shake well. Place chicken and marinade in a heavy-duty zip-top plastic bag, massage marinade into meat for a couple of minutes, then refrigerate for 6 to 24 hours. (You might also want to try this marinade with pork tenderloin or round steak.)

2. Preheat broiler. Spray rack of broiler pan with vegetable cooking spray and arrange chicken on rack. Place rack in

broiler and broil 6 to 8 inches from heat for 15 to 20 minutes, turning occasionally, until cooked through.

Makes 4 servings with 190 calories and 3.8 grams fat each.

Granddaddy Pork Sandwiches

1 pound lean ground pork
½ cup chopped onion
1 8-ounce can low-sodium tomato sauce
1 tablespoon Worcestershire sauce
1 tablespoon brown sugar
1½ teaspoons dry mustard
½ teaspoon freshly ground pepper
1 teaspoon liquid smoke
½ cup Granny Smith apple, chopped fine
1½ cups red cabbage, shredded fine
½ cup pineapple low-fat yogurt
½ cup raw carrot, shredded fine
¾ teaspoon curry powder
6 whole-grain hamburger buns

1. In a nonstick skillet, brown pork over medium heat until it crumbles. Spoon off liquid fat. Remove pork and place on paper towels. Pat off as much fat as possible. Wipe fat from skillet with a paper towel, then return pork to skillet. Over low heat, stir in onion and sauté covered until onion is clear and soft.

2. Add tomato sauce, Worcestershire sauce, brown sugar, 1 teaspoon of the dry mustard, pepper, and liquid smoke, then bring to a boil, cover, reduce heat, and simmer for 15 minutes, stirring occasionally. Set aside, covering it to keep it warm.

3. In a large bowl stir together apple, cabbage, yogurt, carrot, ½ teaspoon of the dry mustard, and curry powder. Serve

immediately by spooning pork mixture evenly onto bottom halves of buns, then topping with cabbage mixture.

Makes 6 servings with 319 calories and 10.8 grams fat each.

London Broil

15 ounces top round steak trimmed of visible fat
½ cup dry red wine
1 clove garlic, chopped fine
Freshly ground black pepper to taste
1 teaspoon dried rosemary, crumbled
Salt to taste

1. Place steak, wine, garlic, and pepper in a gallon-size sealable plastic bag. Massage lightly. Add rosemary and salt, squeeze as much air out of bag as possible, seal bag, turn steak three or four times, then refrigerate for 6 to 24 hours.

2. Remove meat from refrigerator and let sit at room temperature for 30 minutes. Preheat broiler for 20 minutes. Broil 3 inches from heat approximately 4 minutes on each side, turning only once. Allow meat to cool 2 to 3 minutes, then slice thinly across the grain and serve hot.

Makes 4 servings with 176 calories and 4 grams fat each.

Outrageous Chicken Sandwich

1 8-ounce container plain nonfat yogurt
1 teaspoon dried tarragon
1 tablespoon Dijon mustard
¼ teaspoon garlic powder
2 tablespoons lemon juice
4 chicken breast halves (4 ounces each), skinned and boned
4 reduced-calorie whole-wheat hamburger buns, split
4 leaves green- or red-leaf lettuce

4 slices fresh tomato

8 medium-sized canned mild Greek peppers

1. Stir together yogurt, tarragon, mustard, garlic powder, and lemon juice. Place chicken in a heavy-duty zip-top plastic bag, pour in marinade, massage into meat for 1 to 2 minutes, then refrigerate for 6 to 24 hours.

2. Spray rack of broiler pan with vegetable cooking spray. Remove chicken from marinade, place on rack (leave electric oven door partially open), and broil 5½ inches from heat for 6 to 7 minutes on each side or until cooked through.

3. Place lettuce leaves on bottom halves of buns followed by chicken and one tomato slice. Remove stems from Greek peppers and discard. Cut peppers into ¼-inch slices. Arrange pepper slices evenly over tomato slices, then top with remaining bun halves.

Makes 4 servings with 260 calories and 4.8 grams fat each.

Turkey Cheese Loaf

1 tablespoon plus 1 teaspoon olive oil

1 medium onion, chopped

1 pound 4 ounces turkey ground without the skin

½ cup skim milk

3 tablespoons ketchup

1 large egg white, lightly beaten

4 slices day-old whole wheat bread processed into fine crumbs

2 tablespoons grated Parmesan cheese

½ teaspoon ground basil

¼ teaspoon ground thyme

½ teaspoon garlic powder

¼ teaspoon freshly ground black pepper

1. Preheat oven to 350 degrees. Coat an 8″ × 5″ loaf pan with nonstick spray and set aside. Heat oil in a nonstick skillet,

add onion, and sauté over medium heat until tender and clear.

2. In a large bowl stir together cooked onion and remaining ingredients. Form turkey mixture into a loaf and place in coated pan. Bake 50 to 60 minutes until brown and cooked through. Cool 10 minutes and cut into eight slices of equal size.

Makes 8 servings with 181 calories and 9 grams fat each.

Orange and Clove Snapper

1¼ cups orange juice
¼ teaspoon ground cloves
4 red snapper fillets (4 ounces each) about ¾ inch thick
2 teaspoons cornstarch
2 fresh medium oranges, peeled, sectioned, and seeded (about 1 cup)

1. In a small bowl stir together ½ cup of the orange juice and ⅛ teaspoon of the cloves. Coat a 10″ × 6″ × 2″ baking dish with vegetable spray and arrange fillets in dish. Pour orange juice mixture evenly over fillets, cover fillets, and refrigerate for 20 minutes.

2. Preheat oven to 400 degrees. Remove fillets from refrigerator, uncover, and bake for 20 minutes or until fish flakes easily when tested with a fork. Move fillets to a covered serving platter to keep warm.

3. In a non-aluminum saucepan, stir together remaining orange juice and cornstarch. Raise heat to high, bring to a boil, and cook about 1 minute or until mixture has thickened, using a wire whisk. Remove from heat, stir in orange sections and remaining cloves. Spoon evenly over fish and serve.

Makes 4 servings with 174 calories and 1.8 grams fat each.

Savory Rice

½ cup dry white wine
1⅔ cups canned chicken broth
1 cup long-grain rice, uncooked
¼ teaspoon freshly ground pepper
¼ cup finely chopped green onions
1 cup sliced fresh mushrooms
¼ cup finely chopped celery
¾ cup fresh tomato, peeled, seeded, and chopped
¼ teaspoon salt
1 14-ounce can artichoke hearts, drained and chopped
3 tablespoons minced fresh parsley

1. In a medium saucepan stir together wine, chicken broth, rice, and pepper. Bring to a boil, cover, reduce heat, and simmer 20 minutes. Remove from heat and let stand covered for 10 minutes.

2. Coat a large nonstick skillet with vegetable cooking spray and place over medium-high heat until hot. Add onion, mushrooms, and celery, and sauté until tender.

3. Stir in rice from step 1, tomato, salt, artichoke hearts, and parsley. Cover and cook over medium heat for 3 to 4 minutes or until heated through. Serve hot.

Makes 10 half-cup servings with 89 calories and 0.3 gram fat each.

Couscous Casserole

1½ cups water
¼ teaspoon salt
1 cup uncooked couscous
1 8¾-ounce can low-sodium whole-kernel corn, drained
1 15-ounce can black beans, drained
1 7-ounce jar roasted red peppers in water
1 8-ounce can sliced water chestnuts, drained
2 tablespoons pickled jalapeño pepper, minced

⅓ cup minced green onions

2 tablespoons balsamic vinegar

2 teaspoons sesame oil

1 teaspoon ground cumin

1 cup part-skim ricotta cheese

6 cups fresh spinach leaves

1. Preheat oven to 350 degrees. Boil water and salt in a saucepan and remove from heat. Stir in couscous, cover, and let stand 5 minutes or until liquid is absorbed. Stir into couscous corn, beans, red peppers, chestnuts, jalapeño peppers, and onion.

2. Mix vinegar, oil, cumin, and ricotta cheese, then stir into couscous mixture. Lightly coat an 11″ × 7″ × 2″ baking dish with vegetable cooking spray. Spoon mixture into baking dish. Bake uncovered for 25 minutes or until heated through.

3. Slice spinach leaves into thin strips and place 1 cup of spinach on each serving plate. Spoon couscous mixture evenly over spinach and serve.

Makes 6 servings with 299 calories and 5.8 grams fat each.

Shrimp Festival

1 tablespoon plus 1 teaspoon olive oil

1 pound 4 ounces uncooked medium shrimp with tails left on, shelled and deveined

1 tablespoon minced garlic

½ cup dry white wine

¼ cup freshly squeezed lemon juice

½ cup chicken broth

¼ cup minced fresh parsley

¼ teaspoon freshly ground black pepper

¼ teaspoon salt

4 fresh lemon slices for garnish

1. In a medium-sized skillet, heat oil over high heat, add shrimp, and cook, stirring constantly, just until pink (about 2 minutes). While still stirring, add garlic and cook another 30 seconds. Turn heat to low, remove shrimp with slotted spoon, and place shrimp on covered serving platter to keep hot. To same skillet, add wine, lemon juice, chicken broth, parsley, pepper, and salt. Reduce sauce to one-half by returning heat to high and boiling uncovered. Spoon sauce over shrimp and garnish with lemon slices.

Makes 4 servings with 223 calories and 7 grams fat each.

Orange-Lemon Game Hen

2 teaspoons olive oil

1 medium onion, sliced thin and separated into rings

1 medium green bell pepper, cut into strips

2 cups frozen artichoke hearts, thawed

2 tablespoons fresh lemon juice

2 tablespoons chicken broth

4 cloves garlic, cut lengthwise into slivers

1 tablespoon lemon zest (very outside of peel), grated fine

1 tablespoon orange zest, grated fine

½ teaspoon onion powder

1 teaspoon dried thyme

¼ teaspoon freshly ground pepper

¼ teaspoon salt

1 1-pound game hen, skinned and cut in half down the middle

1. Preheat oven to 375 degrees. In a large oven-proof skillet* heat oil over medium-high heat, then add onion and bell pepper. Cook until tender (4–5 minutes), stirring frequently. Add artichoke hearts, lemon juice, chicken broth, and gar-

lic. Raise heat, bring to a boil, and boil for 30 seconds. Remove from heat.

2. In a small bowl combine lemon and orange zest, onion powder, thyme, pepper, and salt. Rub mixture on sides of hen and arrange hen on top of vegetable mixture. Cover and bake for 50 to 60 minutes, or until juices run clear when meat is pricked.

*If you don't have an oven-proof skillet, you can prepare vegetables in a regular skillet, move them to a medium-sized baking dish, place seasoned hen on top of vegetables, and bake according to instructions in step 2.

Makes 2 servings with 319 calories and 12 grams fat each.

Appendix B

The 10-Day Menu Exchange for a Hectic Life

Your boss wants you to spend more time working, your spouse wants you to spend more time alone together, your kids want you to spend more time with them, your friend is having a crisis, your parents and siblings want to see you more often . . . When your life feels as if it's about to explode, or if you just feel lazy and don't want to cook dinner, try this menu exchange. It's the ultimate in simplicity and ease of preparation.

Daily Menus

Day 1

Breakfast

One whole English muffin; 1 tablespoon fruit jam; one slice turkey bacon; half of a grapefruit or one orange.

Lunch

Hot Ham and Cheese Pocket: Inside half of a 6-inch whole-grain pita pocket stuff 2 ounces Canadian bacon, 1 cup raw broccoli florets, and 2 ounces shredded reduced-fat mild cheddar cheese (not to exceed 90 calories per ounce).

Microwave until cheese melts and broccoli is soft. If you don't have a microwave, steam broccoli first, then bake sandwich in oven until cheese melts. Serve with one Granny Smith or other apple.

Snack (anytime)

Stir 1 tablespoon chocolate minimorsels and 1 tablespoon crème de menthe into 1 cup vanilla nonfat yogurt.

Dinner

Healthy Choice Lasagna Roma with Meat Sauce frozen dinner; 2 cups tossed salad topped with 2 tablespoons fat-free salad dressing; one slice French bread topped with 1 tablespoon Fleischmann's 5 Calorie Butter Spread, a sprinkling of garlic powder, and a pinch of basil, then toasted.

Day 2

Breakfast

Two frozen fat-free waffles topped with 1 cup sliced fresh strawberries or peaches dusted with 1 tablespoon powdered sugar; 1 cup skim milk.

Lunch

Turkey Sandwich with Chips: 2 ounces Healthy Choice Oven Roasted Low Fat or other low-fat turkey breast, two regular slices whole-grain bread (not to exceed 70 calories and 1 gram of fat per slice), 1 tablespoon low-fat mayonnaise mixed with a dash of Dijon-style mustard or ketchup, half of a sliced fresh tomato or four to six slices fresh cucumber, freshly ground pepper to taste; 11 Mother's Potato Snaps or other low-fat potato chip (serving should not exceed 2 grams of fat and 60 calories); one yellow or red bell pepper cut into strips.

Snack (anytime)

Double Chocolate Swirl: 12 chocolate Teddy Grahams (teddy bear cookies) dipped in one container Hunts Snack Pack Fat-Free or other fat-free chocolate pudding. If you don't like chocolate, try substituting one container vanilla fat-free pudding.

Dinner

Healthy Choice Traditional Beef Tips frozen dinner; one slice regular whole-grain bread topped with 1 tablespoon lower-fat tub margarine; 1 cup tossed salad topped with 1 tablespoon fat-free salad dressing; 1 cup skim milk; one orange.

Day 3

Breakfast

Three-quarters cup dry high-fiber cereal (choose from Healthy Options Food List in Step 2); 1 cup skim milk; ½ cup orange or grapefruit juice.

Lunch

Roast Beef or Pastrami Sandwich with Cheese Crackers: 2 ounces Healthy Choice or other low-fat roast beef or pastrami luncheon meat, two regular slices whole-grain bread, 1 tablespoon low-fat mayonnaise mixed with a dash of Dijon-style mustard or ketchup, half of a sliced fresh tomato or four to six slices fresh cucumber, freshly ground pepper to

taste; 32 Nabisco SnackWell's Zesty Cheese Crackers; 1 cup
skim milk.

Snack (anytime)

Fruit in Pudding: Dip the tips of 1 cup whole strawberries or
seven dried apricot halves into one 6-ounce container fat-free
chocolate pudding, then eat remaining pudding.

Dinner

Healthy Choice Shrimp and Vegetables Marinara frozen dinner;
one regular slice whole-grain bread topped with 1 tablespoon
lower-fat tub margarine; 2 cups tossed salad topped with
2 tablespoons fat-free salad dressing.

Day 4

Breakfast

Three-quarters cup dry high-fiber cereal; 1 cup skim milk; half
of a banana by itself or sliced and added to cereal.

Lunch

Toasted Ham and Cheese: Toast two regular slices whole-grain
bread, top with 2 ounces Canadian bacon and three slices
Kraft Fat-Free Singles, heat until cheese melts, arrange three
or four thin tomato slices on top of melted cheese, and
sprinkle with optional garlic powder; one medium raw carrot
or stalk of celery.

Snack

New Zealand Fruit Mix (Tip 96).

Dinner

Healthy Choice Sesame Chicken Shanghai frozen dinner; two regular slices whole-grain bread topped with 1 tablespoon lower-fat tub margarine; 2 cups tossed salad topped with 2 tablespoons fat-free salad dressing; one tangerine or orange.

Day 5

Breakfast

One poached egg; one English muffin topped with 1 tablespoon lower-fat tub margarine; 1 cup skim milk.

Lunch

Pita Pizzazz: Toss 2 ounces Healthy Choice Oven Roasted Low Fat or other low-fat turkey breast, ½ cup garbanzo (chickpeas) or other beans, half of a sliced tomato, and 1 cup salad greens with 2 tablespoons fat-free salad dressing, then stuff into half of a 6-inch whole-grain pita pocket.

Snack (anytime)

Sprinkle half of a grapefruit with ½ teaspoon brown sugar and ½ teaspoon apple-pie spice, then broil in oven until sugar melts.

Dinner

Healthy Choice Pasta Shells Marinara frozen dinner; one slice French bread topped with 1 tablespoon Fleischmann's 5 Calorie Butter Spread, a sprinkling of garlic powder, and a pinch of basil, then toasted; 1 cup tossed salad topped with 1 tablespoon fat-free salad dressing; 15 grapes.

Day 6

Breakfast

One cup cooked oatmeal or other hot cereal; 1 cup skim milk; ¾ cup fresh berries.

Lunch

One and one-half servings Progresso Spicy Chicken and Penne Pasta soup with ½ cup cooked pasta added to soup; half of a sliced cucumber soaked for 5 minutes in balsamic vinegar.

Snack (anytime)

One cup fruit-flavored nonfat yogurt.

Dinner

Healthy Choice Chicken Con Queso Burrito frozen food; 2 cups tossed salad topped with 2 tablespoons fat-free salad dressing and either a sixth of a medium avocado, eight ripe olives, or 1½ teaspoons dry roasted sunflower seeds; one regular slice whole-grain bread; 1¼ cups watermelon cubes or two plums.

Day 7

Breakfast

One and one-half cups dry high-fiber cereal; 1 cup skim milk; ½ cup orange or grapefruit juice.

Lunch

Pita Pizzazz: Toss 2 ounces Healthy Choice Oven Roasted Low Fat or other low-fat turkey breast, ½ cup garbanzo (chickpeas) or other beans, half of a sliced tomato, and 1 cup salad greens with 2 tablespoons fat-free salad dressing, then stuff into half of a 6-inch whole-grain pita pocket.

Snack (anytime)

Twelve Keebler Wheatables.

Dinner

Healthy Choice Beef and Peppercorn Cantonese frozen dinner; one regular slice whole-grain bread topped with 1 tablespoon Fleischmann's 5 Calorie Butter Spread; 2 cups tossed salad topped with 2 ounces shredded reduced-fat mild cheddar cheese (no more than 90 calories per ounce) and 2 ounces fat-free salad dressing; one orange.

Day 8

Breakfast

One whole English muffin; 1 tablespoon lower-fat tub margarine; half of a grapefruit or one pear; 1 cup skim milk.

Lunch

Broccoli and Pasta Salad: Toss 1 cup steamed firm broccoli, 1 cup cooked pasta, ½ cup chopped tomato, ½ cup or 2 ounces fat-free mild cheddar cheese, and chopped fresh basil to taste with 2 tablespoons fat-free Italian dressing.

Snack (anytime)

One 6-ounce container fat-free pudding.

Dinner

Healthy Choice Sweet and Sour Chicken frozen dinner; one medium raw carrot or ½ cup steamed carrots; one sliced orange.

Day 9

Breakfast

One whole warm or toasted bagel halved and topped with 1 tablespoon lower-fat tub margarine; 1 cup skim milk.

Lunch

Bacon and Lettuce Sandwich: Two slices turkey bacon, two regular slices plain or toasted whole-grain bread, 1 tablespoon low-fat mayonnaise mixed with a dash of Dijon-style mustard or ketchup, one lettuce leaf, half of a sliced fresh tomato or four to six slices fresh cucumber, ¼ cup raw bean sprouts (optional), freshly ground pepper to taste; one golden delicious or other apple.

Snack (anytime)

Two Nabisco Fat-Free SnackWell's Devil's Food Cookie Cakes; 1 cup skim milk. After you open the stay-fresh cookie package, store them in pairs (two cookie cakes equal one serving) in zip-top sandwich bags out of sight.

Dinner

Healthy Choice Yankee Pot Roast frozen dinner; one regular slice whole-grain bread topped with 1 tablespoon lower-fat tub margarine; 2 cups tossed salad with 2 tablespoons fat-free salad dressing; one orange or nectarine.

Day 10

Breakfast

One whole English muffin topped with 1 tablespoon lower-fat tub margarine; half of a grapefruit or banana; 1 cup skim milk.

Lunch

Chef Salad: 2 cups lettuce, 2 ounces chopped Healthy Choice Oven Roasted Low Fat or other low-fat turkey breast, one-half sliced tomato, one-half sliced cucumber, one-quarter chopped yellow bell pepper, six or so thin carrot shavings using a vegetable peeler, ½ cup bean sprouts, 2 tablespoons fat-free Italian salad dressing; two slices toasted French bread topped with 1 tablespoon lower-fat tub margarine and optional garlic powder.

Snack (anytime)

Combine 1 tablespoon orange marmalade with 1 cup vanilla nonfat yogurt, one sliced fresh peach, and a dash of cinnamon.

Dinner

Healthy Choice Roast Turkey frozen dinner; one regular slice whole-grain bread topped with 1 tablespoon lower-fat tub margarine; 2 cups tossed salad topped with 2 tablespoons fat-free salad dressing.

Appendix C

The Sensible Lifestyle Approach

A common-sense strategy suitable for people who want the most freedom possible during weight loss is the Sensible Lifestyle Approach. You simply use the Healthy Options Food List to guide your food choices while eating the kinds and amounts of food suggested in the Food Guide Pyramid. You'll find both the food list and pyramid in Step 2. Once you've started eating healthy balanced meals, you then perform Steps 5 through 7.

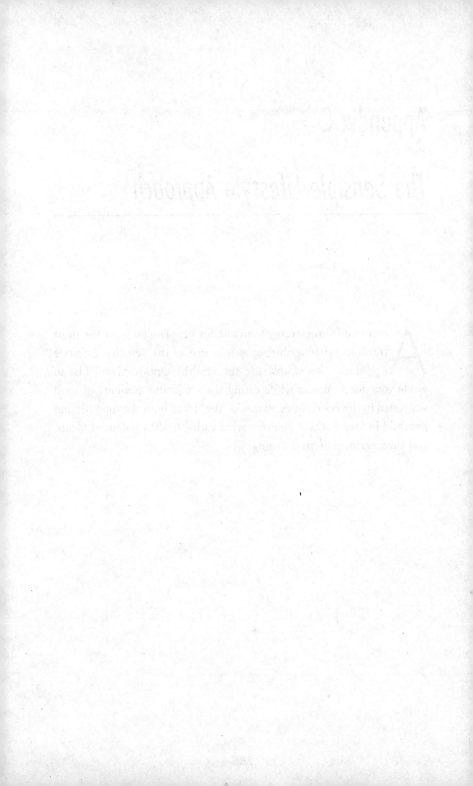

Appendix D

This-Time-It's-for-Real Monitoring Form

How to Use the This-Time-It's-for-Real Monitoring Form

This powerful form will allow you to quickly and easily monitor your food, fitness, and attitudes for a particular day all on one sheet of paper. Looking at the sample form on page 289, you can see that you record the following:

Fitness

- **The activity.** Did you walk, climb stairs, cycle, do housework, play fitness games with kids, lift weights?

- **The time.** Did you try to work out for at least 15 minutes all at one time? If you couldn't, did you try to exercise for 5 minutes at a time three times during the day?

- **How you felt afterward.** Were you sore, depressed, tired, happy, energetic, or maybe relaxed? If you were sore, do you think you should cut back your time by 5 minutes? If you felt great, do you think you should exercise maybe 5 minutes longer next time?

Nutrition

Are you consuming enough servings from the Food Guide Pyramid discussed in Part I? Do you eat too much of one food group and not enough of another? How can you plan your meals better to ensure more balance in your diet?

Food

- **The time you ate.** Look for negative patterns such as eating just before bed, skipping breakfast, or eating late at night.

- **The food and amount.** Do you consistently choose the same foods? What are they? What foods contribute most to your daily calorie goal? Are you eating moderate amounts of food? Are you always aware of how much food you're eating?

- **Your activity while eating.** Were you reading a magazine or newspaper, watching television, or perhaps listening to the radio?

- **How you felt while you ate.** Did you feel bored, angry, lonely, depressed, hostile, jealous, or maybe as if you were celebrating?

- **Calories and fat.** Become aware of the foods you eat that contain the most calories and fat grams, and try to find other foods to substitute for them. Do you feel bad because you lapsed during the week and ate more calories or fat grams one day than you should have? Have you read Tips 994 through 1,000 on lapses?

Make photocopies and
enlarge to desired size.

This-Time-It's-for-Real
Monitoring Form

Fitness

Activity	Minutes	Felt Afterward
_____	____	_____
_____	____	_____
_____	____	_____
_____	____	_____
_____	____	_____

Nutrition

Today's Servings from Food Groups

Milk, Yogurt, Cheese	☐ ☐ ☐
Meat, Poultry, etc.	☐ ☐ ☐
Fruits	☐ ☐ ☐ ☐
Vegetables	☐ ☐ ☐ ☐ ☐
Breads, Cereals, etc.	☐ ☐ ☐ ☐ ☐ ☐ ☐ ☐ ☐

Food

Time	Food and Amount	What You Did While Eating	How You Felt While Eating	Calories	Fat Grams

Total Daily Calories [ ]

Total Daily Fat Grams [ ]

Appendix E

My Realistic Weight-Loss Graph

Make photocopies and
enlarge to desired size.

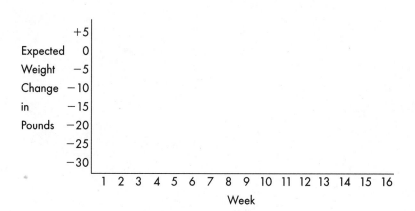

Appendix F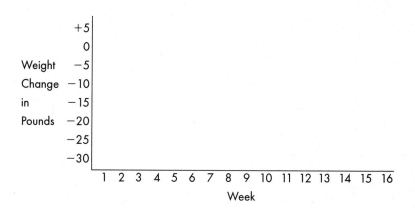

Fat-Attack Graph

Make photocopies and
enlarge to desired size.

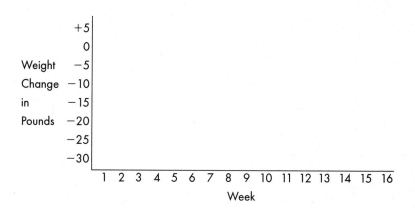

Weight
Change
in
Pounds

+5
0
−5
−10
−15
−20
−25
−30

Week

1 2 3 4 5 6 7 8 9 10 11 12 13 14 15 16

Suggested Readings

The following sources can provide recipes, reinforcement, support, and a more detailed look at some of the themes touched on in this book. This section is divided into periodicals, books, and sources for the North American Weight-Control Survey. Periodicals can be especially helpful because they reinforce your goals each time they arrive.

Periodicals

Food

Better Nutrition for Today's Living, Argus Business, 6151 Powers Ferry Rd., N.W., Atlanta, GA 30339-2941.

Cooking Light: The Magazine of Food and Fitness, 2100 Lakeshore Dr., Birmingham, AL 35209.

Eating Well: The Magazine of Food and Health, Ferry Rd., Charlotte, VT 05445.

Nutrition Action Healthletter, Center for Science in the Public Interest, 1875 Connecticut Ave. N.W., Ste. 300, Washington, DC 20009-5728.

Tufts University Diet & Nutrition Letter, Tufts Graduate School of Nutrition, 53 Park Pl., Floor 8, New York, NY 10007.

Vegetarian Times, 1140 Lake St., Ste. 500, Oak Park, IL 60301.

Aerobic Activities

American Square Dance, Sanborn Enterprises, 661 Middlefield Rd., Salinas, CA 93906-1004.

Backpacker, Rodale Press, 33 E. Minor St., Emmaus, PA 18098-0001.

Bicycling, Rodale Press, 33 E. Minor St., Emmaus, PA 18098-0001.

The Complete Guide to Exercise Videos, Video Exercise Catalog, Dept. EF2, 5390 Main St. N.E., Minneapolis, MN 55421.

Cross Country Skier, 1823 Fremont Ave. South, Minneapolis, MN 55403.

Dance Magazine, Dance Inc., 33 W. 60th St., New York, NY 10023-7990.

Golf, Box 53733, Boulder, CO 80322-3733.

In-Line Skater, 4099 McEwen Dr., Ste. 350, Dallas, TX 75244-5039.

Runner's World, Rodale Press, 33 E. Minor St., Emmaus, PA 18098-0001.

Ski, Times-Mirror Magazines, 2 Park Ave., New York, NY 10016-5675 (aerobic if backcountry skiing).

Snowboarder, Surfer Publications, 33046 Calle Aviador, San Juan Capistrano, CA 92675 (aerobic if backcountry snowboarding).

Speed Skating Times, 2401 N.E. 15th Ter., Pompano, FL 33064 (covers both ice and in-line).

Swim, Swimming World Publications, 228 Nevada St., El Segundo, CA 90245.

Walking Magazine, P.O. Box 52341, Boulder, CO 80321-2341.

Weight Control

Fitness, P.O. Box 3166, Harlan, IA 51593-2357.

Healthy Weight Journal, Hettinger, ND, telephone (701) 567-2845.

Shape, P.O. Box 563, Mt. Morris, IL 61054-7796.

Weight Control Digest, Dallas, TX, telephone (800) 736-7323.

Weight Watchers, Box 56129, Boulder, CO 80322.

Women's Sports and Fitness, 2025 Pearl St., Boulder, CO 80302-4429.

General Health

American Health, 28 W. 23rd St., New York, NY 10010.

Going Bonkers? Harold Publications, 322 Royal Poinciana Plaza, Palm Beach, FL 33480-4094.

Harvard Health Letter, Harvard Medical School Health Publications Group, 164 Longwood Ave., Floor 1, Boston, MA 02115-5818.

Health, P.O. Box 56863, Boulder, CO 80322-6863.

Health and You, Health Corporation, One Executive Dr., Moorestown, NJ 08057-4222.

Health Words for Women, Dawden Publications Company, 110 Summit Ave., Montvale, NJ 07645-1712.

Mayo Clinic Health Letter, Mayo Medical School, 200 First St., S.W., Rochester, MN 55905-0001.

Men's Health, Rodale Press, 33 E. Minor St., Emmaus, PA 18098-0001.

Prevention, Rodale Press, 33 E. Minor St., Emmaus, PA 18098-0001.

University of California at Berkeley Wellness Letter, Healthletter Associates, 632 Broadway, New York, NY 10012-2614.

Books

American Heart Association. *American Heart Association Low-Fat, Low-Cholesterol Cookbook* (New York: Times Books, 1989).

_____. *American Heart Association Cookbook* (5th ed.) (New York: McKay, 1991).

_____. *Brand Name Fat and Cholesterol Counter* (New York: TimesBooks, 1994).

Anderson, B. *Stretching* (Bolinas, CA: Shelter Publications, 1980).

Aslett, D. *500 Terrific Ideas for Cleaning Anything* (New York: Simon and Schuster, 1991).

_____. *Is There Life After Housework?* (Cincinnati: Writer's Digest Books, 1992).

Atlas, N. *American Harvest: Regional Recipes for the Vegetarian Kitchen* (New Paltz, NY: Adam Enterprises, 1991).

Barlow, D. H., and R. M. Rapee. *Mastering Stress: A Lifestyle Approach* (Dallas: American Health Publishing Company, 1991).

Bellerson, K. J. *The Complete and Up-to-Date Fat Book* (Garden City, NY: Avery Publishing, 1993).

Blackburn, G. L., and B. S. Kanders, eds. *Obesity: Pathophysiology, Psychology, and Treatment* (New York: Chapman and Hall, 1995).

Blair, S. N. *Living with Exercise* (Dallas: American Health Publishing Company, 1991).

Brody, J. E. *Jane Brody's Good Food Book: Living the High-Carbohydrate Way* (New York: Bantam, 1987).

————. *Jane Brody's Good Food Gourmet: Recipes & Menus for Delicious Healthful Entertaining* (New York: Bantam, 1992).

————. *Jane Brody's Nutrition Book: A Lifetime Guide to Good Eating for Better Health and Weight Control* (New York: Bantam, 1992).

Brownell, K. D. *The LEARN Program for Weight Control* (Dallas: American Health Publishing Company, 1994).

Brownell, K. D., and J. Rodin. *The Weight Maintenance Survival Guide* (Dallas: American Health Publishing Company, 1990).

Burns, D. E. *The Feeling Good Handbook: Using the New Mood Therapy in Everyday Life* (New York: William Morrow & Company, 1989).

Catalano, E., with W. Webb, J. Walsh, and C. Morin. *Getting to Sleep* (Oakland, CA: New Harbinger Publications, 1990).

Colvin, R. H., and S. B. Olson. *Keeping It Off* (New York: Simon and Schuster, 1985).

Cooking Light magazine. *Cooking Light Cookbook* (Birmingham, AL: Oxmoor House, 1993).

Cooper, K. H. *Kid Fitness: A Complete Shape-Up Program from Birth through High School* (New York: Bantam, 1991).

Cooper, K. H., and M. Cooper. *The New Aerobics for Women* (New York: Bantam, 1988).

Dujovne, C. A., J. Held, G. Peterson, W. S. Harris, and coordinating editor L. Votaw. *A Change of Heart: Steps to Healthy Eating* (Westwood, KS: Professional Nutrition Systems, 1993).

Fletcher, A. M. *Thin for Life: 10 Keys to Success from People Who Have Lost Weight and Kept It Off* (Shelburne, VT: Chapters Publishing, 1994).

Florman, M., and Editors of Consumer Reports. *Fast Foods: Eating In and Eating Out* (New York: Consumer Reports Books, 1990).

Foreyt, J. P., and G. K. Goodrick. *Living without Dieting* (New York: Warner, 1994).

Galvin, J. *The Exercise Habit: Your Personal Road Map to Developing a Lifelong Exercise Commitment* (Champaign, IL: Human Kinetics Publishers, 1992).

Glover, B., and J. Shepherd. *The Family Fitness Handbook* (New York: Penguin, 1989).

Havala, S., and M. Clifford. *Simple, Low-Fat, and Vegetarian: Unbelievably Easy Ways to Reduce the Fat in Your Meals* (Baltimore: The Vegetarian Resource Group, 1994).

Hollis, J. *Fat Is a Family Affair* (New York: HarperCollins, 1985).

Jacobson, M., and S. Fritschner. *The Completely Revised and Updated Fast Food Guide* (New York: Workman, 1991).

Johnson, S. B. *The Walking Handbook* (Dallas: The Cooper Institute for Aerobics Research, 1989). Order from the Cooper Institute for Aerobics Research, 12330 Preston Road, Dallas, TX 75230.

Jones, S. S. *Choose to Live Each Day Fully* (Berkeley, CA: Celestial Arts, 1994).

Josephs, R. *How to Gain an Extra Hour Every Day* (New York: Penguin, 1992).

Kalish, M. *The Dieter's Bible: 375 Ways to Get Thee through the Tough Times* (New York: Penguin, 1992).

Kerr, G. *Graham Kerr's Minimax Cookbook* (New York: Doubleday, 1992).

Kirschenbaum, D. S. *Weight Loss Through Persistence* (Oakland, CA: New Harbinger Publications, 1994).

Kradjian, R. M. *Save Yourself from Breast Cancer* (New York: Berkley Publishing, 1994).

Latella, F. S., W. Conkling, and Editors of Consumer Reports Books. *Get in Shape Stay in Shape* (New York: Consumer Reports Books, 1989).

Martin, R., P. Jamieson, and E. Hiser, eds. *Eating Well Cookbook* (Charlotte, VT: Camden House Publishing, 1991).

Martin, R. A., and E. Y. Poland. *Learning to Change: A Self-Management Approach to Adjustment* (New York: McGraw Hill, 1980).

Mateljan, G. *Cooking Without Fat* (Irwindale, CA: Health Valley Foods, 1992).

McKay, M., and P. Fanning. *Self-Esteem* (2nd ed.) (Oakland, CA: New Harbinger Publications, 1991).

Messina, V. *The No-Cholesterol Vegetarian Barbecue Cookbook* (New York: St. Martin's Press, 1994).

Moran, V. *Get the Fat Out: 501 Simple Ways to Cut the Fat in Any Diet* (New York: Crown, 1994).

National Institutes of Health. *Methods for Voluntary Weight Loss and Control: Technology Assessment Conference Statement* (Bethesda, MD: NIH, 1992). Order from Office of Medical Applications of Research, NIH, Federal Building Room 618, Bethesda, MD 10892.

Natow, A. B., and J. Heslin. *The Supermarket Nutrition Counter* (New York: Pocket Books, 1995).

Netzer, C. T. *The Complete Book of Food Counts* (New York: Dell, 1994).

Ornish, D. *Dr. Dean Ornish's Program for Reversing Heart Disease: The Only System Scientifically Proven to Reverse Heart Disease Without Drugs or Surgery* (New York: Random House, 1990).

_____. *Eat More, Weigh Less: Dr. Dean Ornish's Life Choice Program for Losing Weight Safely While Eating Abundantly* (New York: HarperCollins, 1993).

Oxmoor House Editors. *Cooking Light Cookbook* (Birmingham, AL: Oxmoor House, 1993).

Powter, S. *Food* (New York: Simon and Schuster, 1995).

Rippe, J. M., and P. Amend. *The Exercise Exchange Program* (New York: Simon & Schuster, 1992).

Rodin, J. *Body Traps: Breaking the Binds That Keep You from Feeling Good About Your Body* (New York: William Morrow & Company, 1992).

Rogers, J. *Prevention's Quick and Healthy Low-Fat Cooking* (Emmaus, PA: Rodale Press, 1993).

Rose, N. *Just No Fat: No Fat Cooking with over 400 Recipes of Regular Food for Regular People from Chili Dogs to Cheesecake* (Shawnee Mission, KS: Diets End, 1992).

Salkin, L., and R. Sperry. *365 Ways to Make Love* (New York: Pocket Books, 1996).

Saltzman, J. *Amazing Grains: Creating Vegetarian Main Dishes with Whole Grains* (Tiburon, CA: H. J. Kramer, 1990).

Schlesinger, S. *500 Lowfat and Fat-Free Appetizers, Snacks, and Hors D'oeuvres* (New York: Villard, 1996).

Skinner, J. S. *Body Energy* (Mountain View, CA: Anderson World, 1981).

Stillman, J. *Fast and Low: Easy Recipes for Low-Fat Cuisine* (Boston: Little, Brown and Company, 1985).

Stuart, R. B., and B. Jacobson. *Weight, Sex, and Marriage: A Delicate Balance* (New York: Simon and Schuster, 1987).

Stunkard, A. J., and T. A. Wadden, eds. *Obesity: Theory and Therapy* (2nd ed.) (New York: Raven Press, 1993).

Thoreau, H. D. *Walking* (New York: Penguin, 1995).

Warshaw, H. S. *The Healthy Eater's Guide to Family and Chain Restaurants: What to Eat in over 100 Chains across America* (Minneapolis: Chronimed Publications, 1993).

North American Weight-Control Survey

The Best Place to Start

For convenience, I suggest starting your reading with current or back issues of either *Shape* or *Weight Watchers* magazine. These sources alone contain hundreds of success stories each, with at least three photographically proven stories per issue. Of course all of *Weight Watchers'* stories involve members. If you don't like Weight Watchers, then start with *Shape* magazine. See if your library has current or back issues. If not, then you can order *Shape* back issues by calling (800) 998-0731;

Weight Watchers back issues by calling (800) 876-8441. Other popular and scientific sources are available from the Seattle Institute for Weight Control Research. Send a self-addressed stamped envelope to Seattle Institute for Weight Control Research, Survey Sources, P.O. Box 51015, Seattle, WA 98115.